PROTECTING
THE EMOTIONAL DEVELOPMENT
OF THE ILL CHILD

PROTECTING
THE EMOTIONAL DEVELOPMENT
OF THE ILL CHILD

The Essence
of the Child Life Profession

Evelyn K. Oremland

edited by

Jerome D. Oremland

PSYCHOSOCIAL PRESS
MADISON, CONNECTICUT

Chapter 17 of this volume contains material from "Evelyn K. Oremland's Contributions to the Child Life Profession" by Jerome D. Oremland, M.D., Kim Riemer, M.A., and Albert J. Solnit, M.D. published by Yale University Press in *The Psychoanalytic Study of the Child*, Volume 53, pages 45-50, 1998 and is reprinted here with permission.

Library of Congress Cataloging-in-Publication Data

Protecting the emotional development of the ill child : the essence of
   the child life profession / edited by Evelyn K. and Jerome D.
   Oremland.
       p.   cm.
   Includes bibliographical references and index.
   ISBN 1-887841-20-2
   1. Sick children—Mental health.   2. Sick children—Psychology.
3. Pediatrics—Psychological aspects.   4. Play therapy.
I. Oremland, Evelyn K.   II. Oremland, Jerome D.
RJ47.5.P74   1999
618.92'0001—dc21   99-17720
                                                                CIP

Manufactured in the United States of America

Contents

PART FIVE
The School-Age Child

PART SIX
The Nonhospital Setting

PART SEVEN
A Developmental Model

Preface

Perspectives from Interactions in Pediatric Care

Evelyn K. Oremland, Ph.D.

In writing acknowledgments for this book, foremost have been the efforts of my husband, Jerome D. Oremland, M.D., a psychiatrist and psychoanalyst. I can think back to the many times in the late 1950s when he visited my playroom on the pediatric service at the University of California, San Francisco. Always, he has been readily available for clinical and theoretical consultation, demonstrating his support of my chosen field.

His interest in my work never subsided from delight with what I developed at Mills College, Oakland, California, to encouragement toward the Ph.D. degree I pursued. His support continued as he helped me with contacts and academic contributions on many visits to Israel, India, and Western Europe.

Together in 1973 we edited *The Effects of Hospitalization on Children,* published by Charles C. Thomas. This current book is no exception to his willingness to help, including doing the computer work to ensure that this volume became a reality. Fare-thee-well, faithful friend. It has been an extraordinary relationship.

Our three children must be acknowledged for their help as adults and for what they taught me in their growing-up years. As adults they studied with me at the kitchen table. During their high school years, they never complained about my being elsewhere when I was a graduate student and when I was on the faculty at Mills College. So to Celia Oremland Teter, Noah Oremland, and Annalisa Oremland, thanks for teaching me about children. Thanks, too, for editing help, computer advice, translation of French, and research into mediation on behalf of children and families in California.

To Edna Mitchell, Ph.D., one who is never without a new idea and a well-formulated plan to implement the ideas of others, a special thanks for initiating the Child Life Program at Mills and for maintaining confidence in my competence and leadership, qualities I did not know I had.

To the extraordinary qualities of the Education Department at Mills and especially Jane Bowyer, Ph.D., and Anna Richert, Ph.D., for interpreting the Child Life Program to the campus as a whole. No list of acknowledgments would be complete without mentioning Sharon Smith and Professor Ruth Cossey for what they have done for me.

The Mills College Children's School became a base for my education as well as that of my students. The child-centered philosophy represents a compatibility with the Child Life's dictum of following the child's lead, not operating from an adult's agenda.

My students need to be acknowledged for what they taught me: Because of them, I am much advanced from where I was when I started. I have often thought about how much I did not know at the beginning and have wished I could teach some of the early students again. They taught me what I now know, as is amply illustrated in this volume.

PROTECTING
THE EMOTIONAL DEVELOPMENT
OF THE ILL CHILD

The Play Partnership

There Is More to Know

Evelyn K. Oremland, Ph.D.

Poignancy and drama befall the lives of many children who are ill and hospitalized. Reading accounts of interactions with these child-patients has been my privilege since I began to teach "The Hospitalized Child" course at Mills College. After founding and becoming Director of the Mills College Child Life Program in 1978, I quickly realized that although lectures, seminars, and conferences tell us much, it is only in the journals of our students as they struggle in their internships that we find the essence of the Child Life interaction. This book presents their experiences.

Child Life

Child Life as an approach, a field, and a profession was initially designed to respond to the social and emotional needs

of children experiencing chronic illness and long hospitalization. Playrooms and Child Life Specialists as part of the
architecture and organization of children's hospitals and pediatric units in general hospitals came into being out of
Emma Plank's pioneering work during the 1950s at Cleveland Metropolitan General Hospital (Plank, 1971).

Born in Vienna late in the 19th century, Mrs. Plank studied with Maria Montessori. She became a nursery school
teacher during the time that Anna Freud was applying psychoanalytic theory of development in nursery school programs. Working with Anna Freud, Mrs. Plank's initial work
was strongly influenced by the emerging psychoanalytic understanding of personality development.

Escaping the Nazis, Mrs. Plank and her husband arrived
in the United States in the late 1930s, eventually settling in
California. To increase her credibility as an early childhood
educator and her knowledge of the field in this country,
Mrs. Plank earned a master's degree in child development
at Mills College in 1947.

Quickly established as a leader in early childhood education, in the early 1950s Mrs. Plank was invited to the Cleveland Metropolitan General Hospital. Her initial program was
for children with poliomyelitis and tuberculosis. Recognizing the extraordinary life-adaptations illness required of children, Mrs. Plank extended her approach to all the children
in the hospital evolving new approaches to help these children cope with their circumstances and to minimize the disruptions in development that stem from illness. She
demonstrated that enlightened efforts help maintain the
children's development in the face of the crises and traumas
that characterize their lives. Always, her work was guided
by research that demonstrated the disruption to children's
development by separation and other illness-connected
trauma. From the beginning, reflecting her early experience
with Anna Freud and Maria Montessori, Plank emphasized
the importance of play in any relationship with children (Oremland & Oremland, 1973).

At the Cleveland Metropolitan General Hospital, Plank became the Director of Child Life and Education. It is from her title that Child Life took its name, and her program eventually became the model for Child Life with all hospitalized children. Following her lead, pediatric play programs developed widely in the United States and Canada and throughout much of the Western world, especially England and Sweden (Association for the Care of Children's Health, 1990).

The Child Life field became a profession with the establishment of the Child Life Council of the Association for the Care of Children's Health. The Council specifies principles for the practice of child development-trained personnel who administer play and related therapeutic interventions in pediatric health care settings (Child Life Council, 1989). Hospital fellowships and college-based Child Life programs present education and integrated internships fulfilling the profession's requirements (Child Life Council, Education Committee, 1991). Certification through the Child Life Certifying Commission attests to and maintains the educational and experiential qualities of individual Child Life Specialists.

The Child Life field was further advanced when the American Academy of Pediatrics and the Accreditation Council for Graduate Medical Education, overseeing the training of pediatricians, specified the inclusion of Child Life and related program interventions as standards required in pediatric care (American Academy of Pediatrics, 1990a,b).

Play and Child Life

Research and Child Life

Research consistently supports the value of incorporating psychosocial concerns in children's health care. The effectiveness of Child Life interventions is well documented (Alcock, Feldman, Goodman, McGrath, Park, & Coppelli, 1985; Williams & Powell, 1980).

It is noteworthy that most Child Life research is on the play of children. Whereas the value of children's play is consistently found in every study, research on children's play and Child Life interventions, although informative and academically useful, lacks the necessary detail to enlighten the practitioner about the play partner relationship in Child Life.

The plea for more research on play permeates the Child Life field, especially as the current era of cost containment in health care mounts and threatens to eliminate certain services. Unlike the physical and biological realms, psychosocial considerations do not readily lend themselves to measurement. Realizing that child supportive services are currently not revenue producing, William Sciarillo (1995), Executive Director for the Care of Children's Health, notes that research methods do not adequately capture the worth of Child Life efforts. Richard Thompson (1995) argues that "a broader range of outcome measures [be identified to] indicate success" (p. 11).

Whereas one can only agree with Thompson's and Sciarillo's pleas, it must be remembered that the kind of research best accepted by administrators, that is, quantitative research, is rarely relevant in describing Child Life work. Qualitative studies, essentially case study research, better illustrate the relationship that evolves and develops between the Child Life Specialist and his or her child-patient, and the multiple and often subtle ways in which that relationship maintains the child's ongoing development in spite of disruptive illness and treatment.

Although one may study how play with a host of volunteers and staff differs from play within a consistent and enlightened relationship such as Child Life offers, it will still be difficult to demonstrate the specifics offered by Child Life. Always one must be cautious in that researchers are not immune, nor should they be, from current dominant thinking—cost containment. Without definitive research, the more socially powerful economic interests generally define the debate.

When there is a need to justify the presence of Child Life Specialists one can point to the time Child Life Specialists save nurses and other medical personnel and the reduction in need of medications to quiet children as Child Life Specialists help children participate in rather than resist care. Also frequently forgotten is the "marketing" component to Child Life. Parents uniformly recognize its importance and seek medical settings where it is offered. Nevertheless, it must be acknowledged that times still need to change before administrative eyes can examine and fully understand the implications of the qualitative data of Child Life.

Play Partnerships—The Essence of the Child Life Relationship

In reviewing the writings in Child Life, examples of relationships appear in Plank's (1971) early reports of children, particularly Louis, sometimes called Larry. Larry, a hemophiliac and mentally retarded, was gifted in drawing. Noting his talent, Plank always had art materials and picture books available for him when he was hospitalized. His drawings included numerous depictions related to the hospital and his treatment (Figure 1.1).

Typically, in explaining Child Life, attention is given to describing the purpose of play with children in hospitals and clinics, means of preparing the children for medical–surgical encounters, and consideration of family-centered concerns. Yet to explain the Child Life field requires more than a systematic listing of areas in which professionals interact with children, staff, and families in health care settings.

What frequently happens in the interaction with children depends on the enabling relationship and the support offered in addition to and through play. The importance of

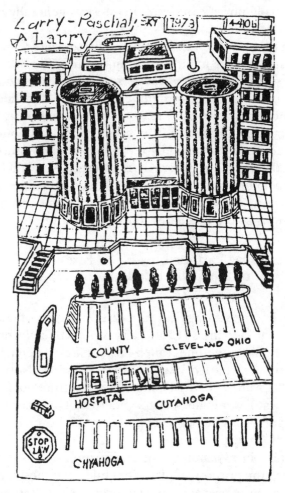

Figure 1.1 The Twin Towers of Cleveland Metropolitan General Hospital. Pen drawing by Larry Paschal (1954–1974)

the relationship in the play partnership is fully documented in students' journals where they report their experiences on various pediatric units. These documents are vivid descriptions of their work and remarkable demonstrations of the ways in which theoretical ideas help understanding. This book emphasizes the qualities in the play relationship that move the child toward mastery of anxieties.

In addition to providing fellow students with stimulating experiences for seminar discussion, the reports of hospital supervisors and related personnel with whom the students work indicate that the Child Life interns in fact promote increased awareness and understanding of children in a wide variety of pediatric professionals. The Child Life interns help staff members pressed by limits of time, budget, and training become aware of the responses of children to illness, injury, hospitalization, and related treatment.

Symbolic Interactionism, Attachment Theory, and Child Life

Child Life uses established theories for its framework. Of particular relevance are symbolic interaction and attachment theory.

It is no longer a surprise that related ideas about human development emerge in separate fields at the same time. Human contexts that shape ideas are influenced by the dominant ideas of an era. At various times factors influence the shift from community-type thinking to thinking focused on the individual—and back again—reflecting parallel political responses. It is no accident that sociological symbolic interactionism and psychological attachment theory arose in the 1960s in attempts to explain relationships.

It was my good fortune to have mentors, colleagues, and friends associated with each of these theories to challenge and encourage me. My chief mentor in sociology, Anselm Strauss, taught the importance of symbolic interactionism, a social psychology first described by George Herbert Mead (1934, 1977) and named and elaborated on by Herbert Blumer (1969).

Mead and Blumer, both keen observers of human behavior, concluded what is now obvious, that on some level humans interact with each other throughout life. Essentially, symbolic interactionism takes note of the nature of the empirical world and the nature of human group life in attempting to explain how individuals respond in small groups. Its premises include that human beings act toward inanimate objects and persons on the basis of the meanings that the objects have.

Blumer explained that meaning is derived from the social interactions one has with one's fellows, emphasizing that human experiences are shaped by earlier human interactions. These meanings are handled in and modified through an interpretive process used by the person as circumstances are encountered. The emphasis on *meanings* becomes central in viewing and understanding play.

Symbolic interactionism helps us understand the play relationship as it develops and is considered over time. It represents a process that forms human conduct. Human beings in interacting with one another have to take account of what each is doing or about to do. Persons respond to others' actions and meanings; the meaning becomes a symbol. People monitor, interpret, and react as they learn the meanings through social interactions. They direct their conduct in terms of what they take into account. Such symbols become readily clear in child development as we watch the children for cues in the play partnerships. One fits one's activity to the actions of others. *It is a conversation of gestures.*

According to Mead, responses are to the meaning of the gestures. When the gestures have the same meaning for two people, each feels understood. Activities are primarily in response to one another or in relation to one another. Human interaction is defined by human activity.

Attachment theory enlightens us regarding the qualities of relationship from the beginning of life, with its near complete dependency, through adulthood with its relative independence (Ainsworth, Blehar, Waters, & Wall, 1978; Bowlby,

1969). Based on empirical research, the variations in a child's attachment behavior illuminate the nature of the child's tie to mother. Particularly in reunion episodes, whether the child maintains proximity and contact or resists and avoids the mother are telling observations with implications for development. The child's diminished playing or lessened vocalizations with "the stranger" with whom he or she is left have important implications for Child Life.

The mother's responsiveness, her acknowledgment of the baby when he or she comes into the room, her affectionate kissing and hugging of the infant, or conversely her inept or routine holding of the infant give us clues as to her part in the dyad. As the infant develops beyond the baby years, his or her smiling or wariness with "strangers," reflecting cognitive acquisitions and social adaptiveness, gives us more to study as we examine the play partnerships characterizing the Child Life relationship.

The synergism of these two approaches was personified for me in my contacts with Strauss and my friendship with psychoanalyst and infant researcher Selma Fraiberg.

As a student, one time I discussed chronic illness in childhood with Strauss. He asked, "But have you learned to think sociologically yet?" My responding pause covered my concern that his question was a gentle affront to the understanding I thought I was expressing. As a good teacher, he guided me to the discovery that there was more to know regarding the social meanings in any context.

With Fraiberg (1980; Fraiberg, Adelson, & Shapiro, 1975), I once discussed an infant–caregiver interaction that had troubled me for its lack of harmony. "Now tell me a story," she responded. My awkward pause reflected that I had already conveyed all I knew about the situation. With extraordinary tact and straightforwardness, Fraiberg showed me that there was more to know if we sought for meaning in what we observed.

Qualitative Analysis

In gathering the student papers and journals for this volume, initially I did not see the exercise as research related. It was Strauss who provided me with lasting encouragement to use students' "data" for studying that which is central to what they do (Glaser, 1967).

Principles in Play Partnerships

Specific principles relevant to work with children in the hospital and clinics are easily evolved from the insights of symbolic interactionism, attachment theory, psychoanalysis, and child development. These principles become the basis for the Child Life play partnerships:

1. The Child Life Specialist's role is explained and/or demonstrated in age-appropriate terms. The Child Life Specialist acts so that the child is clear regarding the professional's role in the adult–child interaction.

2. The Child Life Specialist offers the child play opportunities that the child shapes over time. The child learns that these activities are largely under his or her control.

3. The play partner often focuses on the play as an objective element to interpret as the child allows.

4. As the relationship develops, the Child Life Specialist demonstrates and expresses his or her profound interest in the child and the child's world and experiences. The experience is heightened as connections are made and the Child Life Specialist recalls with the child events previously expressed.

5. The child advocacy role of the Child Life Specialist is patent. As the play partner, the Child Life Specialist represents and interprets the child to the staff members.

6. The Child Life Specialist interprets the context of the illness, the hospital, staff, and treatment to the child and parents.

7. Depending on the child's cognitive abilities, the child may share personal information not shared with anyone else. This sharing of information is seen as a trust that is developing and to be fostered.

8. For children older than 2 years, the Child Life Specialist knows that this play relationship *rarely* substitutes for a primary relationship. For children 2 or younger, prior to establishing object constancy, the play partner often is perceived as the primary caregiver.

9. Always in the forefront of the Child Life Specialist's mind is the fragmenting effects of the multiplicity of relationships that become the child's universe on entering a hospital. The Child Life Specialist knows that he or she is yet another relationship and often but one of a number of play partnerships.

Summary

This book is an invitation to examine the Child Life relationship. The observations are not presented to answer the current call for cost containment in health care institutions. Discouraging as it may seem, research is seldom the basis for change in institutions.

I suggest that the essence of the play partnership in Child Life is not systematically described in existing research. This book presents case studies with children in hospitals and clinics, highlighting the ongoing relationship uniquely offered by Child Life that makes possible a child's progressive psychosocial development despite critical circumstances.

To stimulate further understanding of Child Life, I invited several recent graduates to resubmit their journals to illustrate Child Life case interventions with children in hospitals and in medical–surgical clinics. The descriptions are essentially traditional case study research examples and the data are highly applicable for research. It is my belief that these case studies show the essences of relationship in Child Life play partnerships and as qualitative studies underline the value of those relationships. Although the main focus is on the child in medical care, it should be noted that other fields of child care will recognize similarities to the experiences described and their child-centered interactions are rich with examples of what I have noted here.

References

Ainsworth, M., Blehar, M., Waters, E., & Wall, S. A. (1978). Psychological study of the strange situation. In *Patterns of attachment* (pp. 137–153). Hillsdale, NJ: Erlbaum.

Alcock, D. J., Feldman, W., Goodman, J. T., McGrath, P. J., Park, M., & Coppelli, M. (1985). Environment and waiting behaviors in emergency waiting areas. *Child Health Care, 13,* 174–180.

American Academy of Pediatrics, Accreditation Council. (1990a). *Accreditation manual for hospital, child and adolescent services.* Chicago: Author.

American Academy of Pediatrics, Accreditation Council. (1990b). *Residency review for pediatrics.* Chicago: Author.

Association for the Care of Children's Health. (1990). *North American directory of child life programs.* Bethesda, MD: Author.

Blumer, H. (1969). *Symbolic interactionism: Perspective and method.* Englewood Cliffs, NJ: Prentice-Hall.

Bowlby, J. (1969). *Attachment and loss: Vol. 1. Attachment.* New York: Basic.

Child Life Council. (1989). *Standards for clinical practice.* Bethesda, MD: Author.

Child Life Council, Education Committee. (1991). *Child Life council documents.* Bethesda, MD: Author.

Fraiberg, S. (Ed.). (1980). *Clinical studies in infant mental health: The first year of life.* New York: Basic.

Fraiberg, S., Adelson, E., & Shapiro, V. (1975). Ghosts in the nursery: A psychoanalytic approach to the problems of impaired infant–mother relationships. *Journal of the American Academy of Child Psychiatry, 14,* 387–421.

Glaser, B. G. (1967). *The discovery of grounded theory: Strategies for qualitative research.* Chicago: Aldine.

Mead, G. H. (1934). *Mind, self, and society* (B. G. Glaser & A. Strauss, Eds.). Chicago: University of Chicago Press.

Mead, G. H. (1977). *On social psychology; Selected papers* (A. Strauss, Ed.). Chicago: University of Chicago Press.

Oremland, E. K., & Oremland, J. D. (Eds.). (1973). *The effects of hospitalization on children: Models for their care.* Springfield, IL: Charles C. Thomas.

Plank, E. (1971). *Working with children in hospitals* (2nd ed.). Cleveland: Press of Case Western Reserve University.

Sciarillo, W. (1995). Humanizing health care for children and families: Revitalizing the spirit of our work. *The ACCH Advocate, 2,* 4–8.

Thompson, R. H. (1995). Documenting the value of play for hospitalized children: The challenge of playing the game. *The ACCH Advocate, 2,* 11–18.

Williams, Y. B., & Powell, M. (1980). Documenting the value of supervised play in a pediatric ambulatory care clinic. *Journal of Children's Health Care, 9,* 15–20.

2

The Pediatric Playroom

A Multiple Play
Partners Environment

EVELYN K. OREMLAND, PH.D.

Hospital play programs characteristically involve multiple play partners, individually and in groups, for varying lengths of time, under remarkably differing and extraordinary circumstances. Although play on pediatric hospital units has been described and evaluated in numerous accounts, therapeutic play by Child Life Specialists is essentially an extension of the traditional model of play therapy, the dyad of the

Acknowledgments. The author gratefully acknowledges the help of Susan Marchant who made possible the participant–observation project and the thoughtful, gracious guidance of Maggie Greenblatt whose rich body of information on the children and their situations provided essential context for work in the playroom. Clinical material was provided by Camilla Antoncich, Renee Buonocore, Lisa Cartmell, Sherri Cloward, Tom Collins, Andrea Dezendorf, Gerri Faniel, Lisa Ferczok, Anne Flatley, Rosemary Koefler, Carol Mann, Linda Okazaki, Susan Stern, Janice Yoshikawa, Child Life Specialists, students in Child Life, and nurses.

individual therapist treating an individual child over time (Golden, 1983; Oremland, 1988; Thompson, 1985). Yet the use of play therapy interventions with hospitalized children raises important questions.

The Pediatric Playroom

Although a principal professional such as a Child Life Specialist may administer a play program and be the primary play person for all children on a pediatric unit, a host of staff, including students and volunteers, is involved in play activities with children during any hospitalization. The staff, students, and volunteers all maintain schedules, and rotations occur within the day. Interruptions in play relationships are the norm as medical procedures frequently intercede. Further, although a Child Life Specialist, student, or volunteer may accompany a child to support the child during a procedure, another hospital staff member, probably a nurse or physical therapist, is more likely to treat and be with the child until the child returns to the playroom.

Typically the adult play partner when not accompanying a particular child to the treatment room turns to another child or other children. When the child returns to the playroom from a procedure, sometimes within minutes, sometimes hours later, a new volunteer may have replaced the adult involved in the initial play. The child may play alone or become part of a group supervised by yet another person. Play "emergencies," such as a child's precarious balance on a chair or another's threatening gestures toward a fellow patient, may require the play partner to transfer attention to the problematic child to prevent an accident.

A typical play session in the hospital resembles an "open classroom" or a preschool, but with many differences. A visitor coming to a playroom sees familiar play amidst the bewildering sights and sounds of the hospital. The ages of children participating in one playroom may range from infancy to preadolescence. Most of the children are attached to medical apparatus, most commonly intravenous (IV) tubes carrying medicine-laden fluids from plastic sacks hung on mobile poles. Adults in the room navigate the IV poles for children too young or too disabled to understand that their mobility is dependent on such assistance. The mobility of these IV poles in a sense empowers the children to select where in the room and with what and whom they will play.

For example, in a playroom session five children are attracted to a round table on which a series of doll patients and supplies of alcohol wipes, syringes, tubing, "butterfly" needles, tape, and IV boards used as arm supports are arranged. A Child Life Specialist, Child Life interns, and volunteers seat themselves alongside the children to assist their play. Two 9-year-old girls, concurrently being infused from intravenous connections, thoughtfully treat dolls, replicating their own medical treatment with amazing detail. Three younger boys individually perform various treatments on their "patients," occasionally looking up to observe the activities of others.

At the same time, a boy and a girl, each about 2 years old, balance themselves on their knees on chairs to reach objects in the water table. They experiment with pouring cups full of water onto water wheels. A father of one of the children joins them in the play.

A 3-year-old girl diligently cooks a pretend meal in the child-sized kitchen play area. Next to the windows with a view of the freeway, a 4-year-old boy, whose spastic, neurological disorder renders him unable to walk, delights in pushing miniature cars up a ramp and watching them slide down. A volunteer retrieves them when they go astray.

In a corner, a 5-year-old boy stacks large styrofoam blocks and with wide swinging of his arm that is free of the IV, delights in their crashing to the floor. A volunteer, following the child's directions in the building, supports the play.

Nearby a 9-month-old baby intrigued with a "busy box" is held by his mother. Next to them, a volunteer holds a baby and shakes a rattle to attract the baby's interest. Close by are two 11-year-old boys and a 10-year-old girl playing Monopoly. They argue over the rules of the game and the role of the banker.

Occasionally beeping sounds emanate from the computer-ized control boxes on the IV's, alerting a Child Life Specialist or volunteer to plug in the cord to charge a low battery or to call a nurse to restart infusions. These simple adjustments of medical equipment in the playroom allow play to continue.

During the course of a play session, a pediatric resident enters the room to talk with a child and escorts the child to a treatment room for examination. Medical regimens, never in the playroom, continue throughout the play session with disruptions of play for moments or for hours. Toward noon, with the dispersion of children for lunch, a many times hospitalized 13-year-old boy with cystic fibrosis arrives to plead, "Isn't there a volunteer who can play Monopoly with me?"

When the play session for the afternoon begins, some of the children from the morning session appear alongside new members. Some of the children are acquainted with one another from common experiences in the hospital, previous hospitalizations, and previous visits to the playroom. Generally the Child Life Specialist who coordinates the play and other expressive interventions remains constant, whereas the group of volunteers and several of the student assistants have changed from the morning session.

Multiple Play Partners and Hospital Sociology

The critical fulcrum of therapeutic play is the play relation-ship that in the hospital typically involves multiple play part-ners. Chronically ill children come to know a series of Child

Life Specialists, Child Life students, nurses, volunteers, and other hospital personnel.

A round robin of play relationships is not unique to the pediatric hospital setting (Schaefer, 1976; Schaefer & O'Connor, 1983). All group living arrangements or day care situations involving children require a rotating cast of helping adults (Chehrazi, 1990). Promoting therapeutic play in child care can elevate this care beyond "baby sitting." "Therapeutic Foster Care," labeled by John Murphy and Karen Callaghan (1989), uses models similar to those of Child Life (Hinshelwood & Manning, 1979; Jones, 1976).

Nevertheless, the medical traditions, although influenced by politics and economics, reinforce the development and institutionalization of specialization with its inevitable fragmentation. The introduction and continuing refinement of major technical advances make the modern hospital environment complex and fragmented.

Even though society currently accords greater voice to individuals and their rights and is changing the hierarchical medical world, the potential for fragmentation in medical care is high in the trajectory of any illness event. Although medicine has extended life in ways not even imagined at an earlier time, only the fields related to medicine and nursing, for a variety of social and political reasons, have emphasized concern about individuals and quality of life. This "auxiliary" group, education and mental health professionals, has placed attention on understanding the social and psychological effects of illness and the way patients and families regard the hospital, medical professionals, and medical–surgical treatment (Strauss & Glaser, 1975).

Even though pediatric departments have recently incorporated Child Life Specialists and education and mental health professionals in their organizations, nonmedical services, although important, are secondary. The fact is that children are not admitted to the hospital for play programs.

Mental health professionals and Child Life Specialists view their approaches as advocates for the individual and the family and a corrective to the inevitable fragmentation characteristic of the modern hospital. However, it is important to examine whether play relationships and related interactions are contrafragmenting or if they replicate the fragmentation characteristic of the institutions in which these nonmedical services are embedded. In short we must question whether the disparate therapeutic play relationships characteristic of the hospital add confusion rather than integration and consolidation of experiences for children, an articulated goal of therapeutic play.

It is important to identify the therapeutic processes at work when multiple caregivers engage in play interactions with the children. Easily identified within these complex play systems are countless expressions of development-supportive play comingled with abreactive–cathartic play in the context of the multiple play partners. An ideal place to study the varieties of therapeutic play with multiple caregivers within changing contexts is the pediatric hospital playroom.

Therapeutic Play

The hospital playroom is alive with varieties of play much of which is best regarded as therapeutic play rather than play therapy. *Therapeutic play* primarily provides opportunities for the children to engage in development-supportive and abreactive–cathartic activities.

Development-supportive play refers to those multitude of learning experiences about the developing emotional and physical self and its relation to others that manifest themselves in children's play. Development-supportive activities include providing fine motor practice, general cognitive advances, and social development. Small children refine skills through manipulating play materials; older children try out social roles with peers and adults. These vital activities support and encourage social, psychological, and educational progressions that help offset the high potential of critical health care experiences to disrupt development. Pari parsu therapeutic play allows the development of supportive peer and adult relationships to help children make sense of their current medical crises and assist them in mastering the associated anxieties.

Abreactive–cathartic play encompasses expressive enactments related to conscious and unconscious reliving of ongoing and past traumatic experiences. In abreactive–cathartic play alloplastic trauma is transformed into autoplastic triumph. The therapeutic dimension in abreactive–cathartic play is enlarged by the play partner's interpretations of the play activity, that is, by the play partner's putting into words difficult to express ideas and feelings. Educated guesses at meanings enable the child to maintain expressive interactions in the play and have feelings validated.

The most dramatic form of abreactive–cathartic play is *medical play.* The making active of that which has been experienced passively is seldom enacted as patently as in the medical play in pediatric playrooms (Oremland, 1988; Waelder, 1932). Even casual observation of the children's intense involvement with medical play, as they "treat" doll patients, fellow patients, staff, and themselves with medical equipment and toy versions of medical–surgical apparatus from giving injections to body casting, often with minute replication, reveals their attempts actively to master the traumatic experiences that they must submit to passively that characterize hospitalization and medical–surgical treatment (Figure 2.1)[1]

---

[1]It is controversial as to whether children should be allowed to "treat" fellow patients and staff. Many experts feel that "hurting" a real person can unduly frighten the child and that it is better that the play always be "treating" dolls.

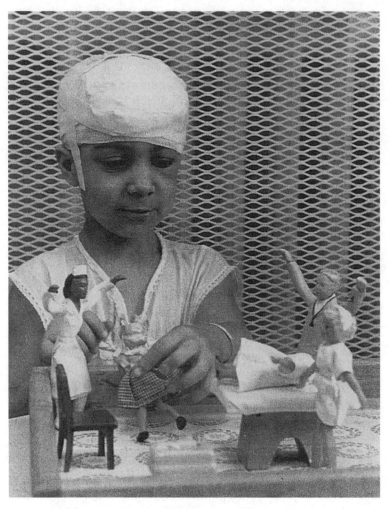

FIGURE 2.1 Medical Play

The integrally related nature of the child's circumstances renders any separation of "outside" and "inside" issues artificial, exaggerating for the Child Life Specialist the dilemmas inherent in therapeutic play. The short-term nature of most hospitalizations often requires the Child Life Specialist to work without full understanding of the "outside" problems, even though a child's play may be rife with the complicated issues related to difficult social and psychological situations, compounded by illness and treatment, that are common to many sick children.

The focus of *therapeutic play* in contrast to *play therapy* is on the promotion of continuing "normal development" and the enabling of children to respond more effectively to their health care experience. Therapeutic play is play that is development-supportive comingled in pediatric play relationships with abreactive–cathartic enactments related to illness and hospitalization issues. *Therapeutic play does not have as its primary goal personality change and is distinct from play therapy.* Whereas *play therapy* addresses basic and persistent difficulties in a patient's interactions in his or her world and generally occurs in the context of a continuity person, *therapeutic play* in a less structured way focuses on spontaneous phenomena as the child engages in play to aid mastery of developmental challenges and current critical events.

The Play Relationships

Cases taken from the journals of selected Child Life students demonstrate that even with a multiplicity of play partners, comingled development-supportive and abreactive–cathartic play, therapeutic play occurs with obvious amelioration of acute and prolonged serious difficulties. These changes in behavior reflect the "self-healing" nature of play noted by Erik Erikson (1950). More precisely, as the child's feeling of being in control is facilitated through supportive play relationships, his or her sense of mastery is enhanced (Bolig,

Fernie, & Klein, 1986). However with striking frequency, especially in severe circumstances, the importance of the child's "selecting" a particular adult, in our cases a Child Life student, and the student's capacity to respond, become the key agents in the often dramatic changes.

These children avidly grasp play opportunities and organize them according to their experiences (Erikson, 1950). Their play, often a condensation of the confluence of their experiences, provides extraordinary opportunities for mastery of anxieties. The tendency of children to "select" an adult places an unusual responsibility on the adult sponsors of the play environment and on those involved in their care and treatment. In every interaction important opportunities are easily overlooked and lost.

The Ideal

That the hospital and its personnel become part of the ongoing lives of the chronically ill child is obvious. The data require that we evaluate the benefits and limitations of these multiple and changing relationships. The children's development, influenced by their illnesses and the treatments, is integrally related to the interactions with the host of caregivers over time. The support for the children's development becomes a mandate for the entire staff.

Although the environment in which Child Life operates reflects the many integrated facets of the hospital complex, nonillness issues arising in play provide the potential and challenge for play therapy. Specific assignments for the army of play associates should emphasize continuities. Sharing of information and developing a consensus among the caregivers, both medical and nonmedical, regarding a unified and integrated series of goals are achievable ideals.

Accurate records of interactions of children, including their play, must be conveyed to successive Child Life Specialists and to the general staff. Reporting to the hospital agencies and those outside its walls that are involved in the care, especially of younger children, informs these groups about approaches that can be continued. Contact with schools is essential if educational development and peer group experiences are to continue.

"Holistic" ideas currently inferred relative to all aspects of children's care cross-sectionally need to be complemented with the longitudinal perspective. A model for ongoing psychiatric consultation for Child Life Specialists was developed by the Child Life "team" at Bellevue Hospital, New York (Wotasik, Mattsson, Longman, & Lewis, 1985).

What is required is systematic evaluation of how children perceive multiple caregivers and multiple play partners. Even when the multipersonnel approach tries to follow a unified approach, attention to coordination of the concomitant and sequential roles only partly ameliorates the complications of the multiple play relationships.

The question remains: Does the unified approach potentially lead to confusion as the continuous relationship is blurred by the numerous caregivers and play partners sharing responsibilities and roles? We know that frequently in group care for young children a child "selects" from the multiple caregivers a particular caregiver with whom the child engages in consistent interaction including play (Stevens, 1980).

Clearly the most effective use of multiple caregiving in the health care environment comes when an effective parent takes on the chief coordinating role. Working with parents to help them strengthen their role when need be is an essential Child Life task. Training and ongoing instruction for volunteers is essential if all interactions are to been seen as opportunities for therapeutic play. To the extent that these recommendations can be effected, the problematic and inevitable multiple caregiving environment can reach higher levels of coordinated efficiency.

Children generally experience multiple caregivers, potential play partners, throughout their formative years. Day care and schools are prime examples of institutions in which children are introduced to multiple relationships. Even though children are resilient, it is suggested that the ideas presented here, applicable beyond the health care world, serve as cautionary notes for multiadult helping relationships in order that fragmentation be minimized.

References

Bolig, R., Fernie, D., & Klein, E. (1986). Unstructured play in hospital settings: An internal locus of control rationale. *Children's Health Care, 15,* 101–107.

Chehrazi, S. (Ed.). (1990). *Psychosocial issues in day care.* Washington, DC: American Psychiatric Press.

Children's Health Care (1988). Play in health care settings. Special issue. *Children's Health Care, 16.*

Erikson, E. (1950). *Childhood and society.* New York: Norton.

Golden, D. (1983). Play therapy for hospitalized children. In C. Schaefer & K. O'Connor (Eds.), *Handbook of play therapy,* (pp. 213–233). New York: Wiley.

Hinshelwood, R. D., & Manning, N. (Eds.). (1979). *Therapeutic communities: Reflection and progress.* London: Routledge, Kegan Paul.

Jones, M. (1976). *Maturation of the therapeutic community.* New York: Human Sciences Press.

Murphy, J., & Callaghan, K. (1989). Therapeutic versus traditional foster care: Theoretical and practical distinctions. *Adolescence, 24,* 891–900.

Oremland, E. (1988). Mastering developmental and critical experiences through play and other expressive behaviors in childhood. *Children's Health Care, 16,* 150–156.

Schaefer, C. (Ed.). (1976). *Therapeutic use of child's play.* New York: Jason Aronson.

Schaefer, C., & O'Connor, K. (Eds.). (1983). *Handbook of play therapy.* New York: Wiley.

Stevens, A. (1980). *Infant psychiatry.* Conference presentation. University of California, San Francisco.

Strauss, A., & Glaser, B. (1975). *Chronic illness and the quality of life.* St. Louis: C. V. Mosby.

Thompson, R. (1985). *Psychosocial research on pediatric hospitalization and health care.* Springfield, IL: Charles C. Thomas.

Waelder, R. (1932). The psychoanalytic theory of play. *Psychoanalytic Quarterly, 2,* 208–224.

Wotasik, S., Mattsson, A., Longman, C., & Lewis, N. (1985). *An interdisciplinary model to extend the Child Life role in the care of families in crisis.* Presented to the Association for the Care of Children's Health, Boston.

Part One

Child Life and Extended Complex Hospitalizations

3

Charlie

A 23-Month-Old
Burned Child

KELLY IRENE NOTTINGHAM

Charlie, a 23-month-old, had been hospitalized since he was 6 months old after being trapped in a burning house during a fire that took the lives of two of his siblings. Charlie's surviving sibling, a 4-year-old sister, was also severely burned.

Charlie suffered third-degree burns over 70% of his body. Only his back, the top of his head, and the palm and fingers of his right hand were spared. Charlie has undergone numerous skin grafts to repair his wounds. Until recently he had a tracheotomy to assist his breathing, which had been compromised by smoke inhalation and heat. He has undergone multiple reconstructive surgeries to build ears, a rudimentary nose, eyelids, and lips. He periodically undergoes "release procedures" to protect his new grafts and to prevent strictures webbing and inappropriate graft growth patterns.

Charlie is often placed in various braces of rigid plastic casts, dressings, and an airplane splint, a brace that forces the child's arms out from the sides of the body at shoulder height. Due to his new skin grafts, he is sometimes confined to bed rest or may be placed in a sitting position in a special chair in his playpen. Occasionally he may be free of most of his braces and can be carried, rocked, and held. Charlie has excellent head control but has not had the opportunity to develop much torso strength. He has never crawled or walked because of the restrictions imposed on him by his grafts. He is able to grasp objects in his right hand with some limited control. His left hand is usually bandaged.

After the fire, the court severed the parental custody rights for Charlie and his sister. The parents, who have a history of drug addiction, were unavailable to provide medical or developmental history about Charlie, are divorced, and have never visited Charlie in the hospital. Charlie's sister was admitted to a different hospital. The two siblings have not seen each other since the fire. No extended family has been identified. The current plan is to reunite the children in a foster care placement.

Charlie is cared for by a large and diverse team of specialists, including doctors, nurses, a speech therapist, a physical therapist, an occupational therapist (OT), a social worker, and personal care assistants. Charlie is discussed regularly on "rehab" social work rounds. Charlie has bedside visits from Child Life volunteers and has been able to accompany them to the playroom for short visits.

Charlie recently began self-induced vomiting by sticking his finger down his throat. His periodic refusal to eat and self-induced vomiting cause the staff great concern. The nursing staff's response varies greatly, ranging from a matter-of-fact quick clean-up without discussion, to a frustrated, angry "bawling out," to expressions of concern with an effort to identify the precipitating event.

The vomiting incidents, which may occur once or twice a day, do not seem to be related to a particular interaction with a caregiver or a common experience. However, I have observed Charlie's reaching for his mouth when he has been left for more than 20 minutes in his playpen chair without direct adult attention. At these times I have been able to distract him by changing the toys in his immediate area and by talking with him. I wonder if it would help to assign a primary caregiver for feeding activities. At the moment, the main "treatment" is a feeding tube placed directly into his stomach through the abdominal wall to keep him hydrated.

Assessment

Charlie is an alert, engaging, generally cheerful toddler. He hears and sees well. He tracks objects with his eyes and recognizes favorite toys. He can vocalize, making an excited sound, a cry, and a persistent clicking sound. He also makes a type of "raspberry" sound. He has limited facial mobility but demonstrates delight by squinting his eyes and making a gurgling sound. He also has a straightforward laugh. He actively explores his environment visually and manipulates toys physically to the extent he is able. Charlie enjoys the attention of adults, making good eye contact, and mirroring some of their movements and the rhythm of their speech. He has not yet used words. There is a quality to Charlie that draws adults to him. He responds eagerly to most adults by reaching out to them or giggling when they smile and say his name. He is deluged with well-wishers who briefly stop by his crib, greet him, and move on.

Charlie is usually cooperative with his caregivers. He rarely becomes upset, although he cries, twists away, and thrashes when he is put in bed restraints to prevent his scratching itchy grafts and when wound dressings are changed. Staff members use distractions such as singing to him and stroking his hair to soothe him.

Although Charlie's abilities in every area have been delayed or restricted by his injuries and the experiential limitations of his life in the hospital, I have made several informal assessments of Charlie's development using the Denver II Developmental Screening Test. Between graft cycles, and if well rested, Charlie consistently scores at the 12- to 13-month level in personal social skills, failing only the "feeds self" item, an impossible task with his impairments. In fine motor adaptive skills, Charlie scores at the 5-month level. He scores at the 4-month level in gross motor skills. Charlie's current speech capacities are those of a 5- to 6-month-old infant.

Aside from the relationships that have evolved with an occupational therapist and me, Charlie has not had the opportunity to develop a significant attachment to any consistent, responsive caregiver. He shows a change in body posture in recognition of my presence, as well as a generally cheerful disposition when I visit. He behaves similarly with the OT.

Social and Environmental Contexts

When confined to bed Charlie watches TV, although he has no control over volume or program. He also can manipulate various toys hung in front of him. Charlie has had little interaction with other children in the rehab unit, most of whom are older and are either paraplegic and/or brain injured. The rehab unit is generally kept darkened with people tending to speak in hushed voices. Charlie is the only burn patient in the unit. His physical appearance is disturbing to some of the children. I have witnessed a few children averting their eyes when passing him or grimacing when they view him. Charlie gives no outward sign that he notices their reactions and continues to smile and try to engage them with his eyes. Not to upset the other patients and their families and "to give Charlie some privacy," the nurses often separate him from the view of the others by a half-pulled curtain around his high crib, further isolating him and preventing him from social interactions.

When Charlie is in his playpen, his visual radius is restricted to the undersides of two rows of beds and a partial view of the hall. The rehab unit is crowded, and the nurses constantly squeeze past Charlie's playpen to reach the equipment lockers and supplies. Due to space constraints, Charlie's playpen cannot be brought into the playroom. He can visit the playroom by being carried or wheeled in a chair. The children in the playroom, mostly hematology and oncology patients, tend to ignore Charlie. Occasionally one asks why he looks different. Charlie watches them with interest as they play but focuses mostly on the adults or the manipulative toys within his reach.

With rare exceptions, Charlie is compliant and alert enough to be examined and treated. Although the scheduling of various occupational and speech therapists is somewhat flexible, it is not designed to accommodate changes in Charlie's mood or energy level. The visits by his three therapists, who are charged with assessing and addressing his physical and developmental impairments, require him to attempt specific tasks and exercises. The pace of these activities is defined by the adults who have only a brief time to achieve maximum results from the prescribed interventions.

Charlie does not appear upset by changes in caregiving personnel. He may reach toward people and return hugs. He is able to discriminate among his caregivers and associate them with previous experiences. When he sees me, he reaches out to play patty cake, a game I often play with him. His body tenses when physiotherapists, who have recently caused him pain during dressing changes, appear at his bedside. Charlie has had many volunteers in his hospital life, almost all of whom have changed over time. Those who work with him are frequently rotated in and out of the rehab unit and often work unpredictable and part-time shifts.

Charlie's most consistent caregiver has been his occupational therapist, who has seen him 5 days a week, an hour per visit, over the past year. Besides range of motion exercises, her interventions include making molds for the plastic braces and graft guards he must periodically wear. She is usually involved in dressing changes related to his grafts. Many of these procedures are difficult and painful for Charlie.

The occupational therapist is sensitive to Charlie and knows how to calm him when he is upset. She has genuine affection for him. She sings songs to him and tells him everything she is going to do before she does it. Charlie responds with smiles and gurgles.

Even though he often has his most intense pain and rages when she is performing a painful procedure with him, she is his primary caregiver. She acknowledges his feelings, attempts to calm him, and engages him in a pleasurable activity at the end of each procedure.

Child Life Interactions with Charlie

Because of his young age and severe disabilities I have listed the Child Life principles that seem most applicable to my work with Charlie:

1. I try to respond consistently to Charlie's vocal and physical cues and signs of distress.

2. I pace activities according to his cues, respecting his need to engage and disengage in activities, and reinforcing his sense of being an individual. Through empathic nurturance, I attempt to reflect and validate his feelings when he is upset.

3. I make frequent and meaningful eye contact to further Charlie's sense of connectedness, self-worth, and recognition that he is a unique individual.

4. I hold him tenderly and gently stroke his uninjured skin, which he enjoys.

5. I provide him with language-rich interactions by naming objects and actions and expanding meaning through empathic interpretations.

6. I provide Charlie with choices of materials and actions to further his sense of affecting his environment.

7. I engage him in interactive games such as peek-a-boo and patty cake to further a sense of intimacy and partnership.

8. I encourage play opportunities to facilitate his continuing development.

9. To the extent possible, I provide a predictable, scheduled playtime with him to develop a sense of being trustworthy and consistent.

10. I encourage his other caregivers to provide him with play opportunities during times I am unavailable to him.

Initiating Child Life Work with Charlie

In the beginning, I had a nurse with whom Charlie was familiar bring me to his bedside. For the next week I visited him twice a day. Each visit was 5 to 60 minutes, depending on Charlie's cues. With each visit I brought a familiar and a novel manipulative toy. I wanted to allow Charlie to gain mastery by successfully manipulating a familiar toy and then enlarge his scope by using a novel object. I sang simple songs, taught him patty cake, and played peek-a-boo games.

Charlie enjoyed our interactions and responded with a gleeful laugh and many smiles. I warned Charlie in advance of my departure, and we made a game of playing patty cake "one last time" before I left. As Charlie and I became more "in tune" with each other, he initiated several of our reciprocal games such as peek-a-boo, a sign that our relationship was progressing.

When Charlie was physically able, I arranged that he visit the playroom. I wanted to introduce Charlie to observations of and interaction with other children. In my journal, I noted:

> I know that Charlie spends most of his waking hours in the rehab ward, which is much quieter and darker than the playroom. In rehab he is protected and isolated from other children. I enlisted the help of a male volunteer, of whom Charlie is fond, to bring Charlie to the playroom.
>
> We used his stroller-type wheelchair and had permission to carry him on a clean sheet. Because of his grafts, no water play or messy art was permitted.
>
> I wanted Charlie to assimilate the new stimuli. We started by wheeling him along the windows that looked into the playroom and by slowly passing the open door. We described what the kids were doing and named some of the toys. We made reassuring and encouraging comments. Charlie was alert, and his gaze flitted all over the room. In that he did not appear to be anxious, we transferred him to the male volunteer's arms and positioned him so that he could look over his shoulder. This allowed Charlie a bird's eye view of activities. We didn't want him to be overwhelmed by being laid on a mat in the center of the fray.
>
> I kept a close watch on him, talking to him about what he was seeing. Charlie's face lacks the ability to show much emotion due to the extensive scarring. I paid attention to Charlie's body language and eye movements to gauge his comfort–anxiety level. He held tightly to the volunteer and visually checked me frequently. He began to gurgle and smile. After a few minutes we moved Charlie to the mat in a seated position. With the volunteer providing needed postural stability I sat in front of Charlie and played with him. My intent was to balance Charlie's need for stimulation and socialization with his need for physical and emotional safety. Interestingly, none of the children interacted with Charlie or asked about his diagnosis or treatment as they often do with new children. Perhaps this was because of his unusual appearance.

Charlie enjoyed playing with the "busy box" I provided. Although hampered by thickly bandaged hands, for 15 minutes he manipulated the toy's many dials, knobs, and changing images. Charlie has few things that he can control in his life. He was truly joyous when using the busy box especially when he could make it make a noise. After a few more minutes of play Charlie began to show signs of being tired, and we escorted him back to his room.

Child Life and Charlie's Caretaking Team

An important way to advocate for a child is to become a trusted and contributing member of the child's caregiving team—which means establishing a rapport with the other professionals who are involved with the child's care. An example from my journal illustrates this point:

The next week I visited Charlie at his bedside. He was a bit groggy from a morphine injection that had been given in preparation for a dressing change. A student nurse arrived to take his vital signs. The student nurse explained that he was "going to be in hot water" with his supervisor if he didn't get them.

Charlie was half asleep and began to swat at the student nurse and howl. The student nurse emphasized the importance of getting the signs prior to the dressing change. I asked the nurse to give me a minute alone with Charlie to calm him down. I gently talked to Charlie, who seemed to recognize my voice. I told him that I understood he just wanted to sleep and be left alone right now. I told him that the nurse would be back in a minute and what the nurse would do. I stroked Charlie's head and spoke quietly and reassuringly. Charlie calmed down immediately.

When the nurse returned I talked Charlie through the procedure, which was brief and noninvasive. The nurse was pleased, and Charlie and I visited before he drifted off to sleep. It was clear that the nurse was going to do the exam in spite of Charlie's protest. By giving both Charlie and the nurse a chance to prepare for the interaction, the encounter became calmer and supportive.

Another example involves Charlie's OT:

Charlie had an extremely painful procedure that required leaving large open wounds that were to be grafted later. Charlie had gone through a horrific experience in the morning with a team of several doctors changing his dressing. That procedure had taken much longer than expected, and both Charlie and the team had been emotionally exhausted afterward.

I enter the room to check on Charlie. He was receiving medications through his gastric tube and is on oxygen. He appeared "spent" both emotionally and physically. His OT approaches with a large casting tray and several splints for Charlie's hand and legs. Before she can say a word, Charlie starts screaming and thrashing. She informs me that she was part of the morning team and that Charlie understands what is coming. She does her best to calm and reassure him. I offer to help by soothing and coaching him through the procedure while she changes his dressings and fits him with the new splints. She says she would appreciate the help. She is upset that she is not allowed to give Charlie any more pain medication before we start.

The procedure lasts almost 2 hours. Charlie is obviously exhausted and in great pain with each manipulation of his limbs. Together, the OT and I talk Charlie through it, frequently allowing Charlie to compose himself. It is frustrating for all of us. When it is over, we wash up and return to play with Charlie. He seems relieved to have control again and after a while begins laughing.

Charlie's Future

Charlie will be hospitalized into the foreseeable future. The hospital is his entire world. Until a foster care parent is assigned to become part of his life, the hospital staff is his family.

In planning for Charlie, the following should be considered:

1. Charlie requires a consistent, responsive caregiver to establish secure attachments.

2. A psychiatric evaluation of Charlie's feeding problems should be initiated.

3. The interdisciplinary team should develop and implement a plan for meeting Charlie's psychosocial needs including being sensitive and responsive to his cues. An inservice should be given to caregiving staff and volunteers on the issue of attachment relative to multiple caregivers, the importance of secure attachment as a developmental milestone, and the significance of attachment in promoting subsequent development.

4. The team should advocate for a foster parent to be assigned as soon as possible to begin regular, consistent visits. The foster parent should receive information on Charlie's communication style and preferences in caregiving. Play and physical contact should be encouraged as a basis for the relationship.

5. Until such time as a foster parent can be assigned, a "foster grandparent" or committed volunteer who is available on a daily basis should be assigned to Charlie.

6. As frequently as possible, Charlie should be taken to the playroom for social interactions and play that will facilitate his cognitive and language development. Emphasis should be placed on activities in which Charlie affects his environment. Whenever medically feasible, Charlie should be given opportunities for water play, painting, and other process-oriented creative activities. He should have a responsive adult present who can aid him in communicating with other children.

7. A language-rich atmosphere should be created, to assist Charlie in associating names with objects and to describe and interpret his interactions with the people and materials around him. The use of puppets, reciprocal chants, and simple games would be beneficial.

8. Visits to Charlie's bedside need to be better controlled by developing a set of guidelines. He needs quality not quantity interaction. A unified philosophical approach toward

meeting his socioemotional needs should be articulated and communicated to those who interact with Charlie, especially the volunteers. Reminders might be posted at bedside.

9. Charlie's crib environment should be monitored in terms of optimal stimulation and opportunities for play. Toys to which he is attached should remain and others rotated. Television should be limited. Attention should be paid to Charlie's visual field, and opportunities for positive visual interaction should be considered when placing him in his playpen.

10. The observations of Child Life staff and volunteers should be recorded in an informal log that could be kept at Charlie's bedside to inform his numerous caregivers of his progress and achievements as well as concerns. The availability of a log might lead to greater consistency in caregiving. Subtle changes of mood or demeanor and successful strategies should be documented. This approach may serve to heighten the awareness of the caregivers to the importance of their social interactions with Charlie. The log could be used as an ongoing resource for discussion at rounds and provide a sense of Charlie's history for his future foster family.

Joel

A 22-Month-Old Abused Child

Rebecca J. Rice

Injury from an unknown perpetrator sent 22-month-old Joel to the Intensive Care Unit (ICU) for 6 weeks. He was then admitted to the pediatric ward, where I met this seriously ill toddler. Joel's father is in jail on a "bad checks" charge. His mother has visited him only once and when she came, Joel screamed and screamed. He has had visitors only one other time while I have been at Children's Hospital. He has no "circle of safety."

Assessment

The first time I saw Joel he was quietly lying flat on his back in his bed. Fully restrained, he was looking up at the television. His large intestine was in a "Zip-Loc" bag for healing and drainage. He was connected to many tubes for drainage of his stomach and gall bladder. A Broviac was installed for infusion on liquids and lipids. He had large abdominal dressings covering the "Zip-Loc" bag with its unbelievable contents. His physical condition must have caused him great stress and anxiety, yet I saw an inactive and silent young child. Behind all the dressings and tubes, I observed a smiling, beautiful child with warm brown skin tones, a full head of richly colored brown hair, and engaging sparkling brown eyes. I was to be the primary Child Life person working with Joel, meeting with him a part of each morning 4 days a week. At this time, Joel could say only "No, No," which was the product name of his arm restraints. His primary language might be Spanish. Most days when I visited Joel, he was in bed with the TV, mounted high on the wall, his only company. Joel occasionally looked up at the TV when the scene changed. His crib with the plastic restraining enclosures is sparsely decorated with a photo of Joel and possibly his sister (no one seems to know for certain), a religious card, and one stuffed animal sitting in the corner that Joel cannot see or reach.

Initially, all I could do was to talk with him about looking away or not moving when procedures were in progress. I planned to be with him, hold his hand, talk and sing during procedures, blow bubbles, and tell him stories.

Because Joel was entirely dependent on others for his care, I wanted to help him gain some sense of autonomy. I decided to encourage him to name and show me medical objects. I would respond by telling him about their use. Gradually I introduced Joel to medical materials specific to his experience.

I wanted to further his understanding of his injuries. Even though Joel was a victim of abuse, I did not want him to feel at fault for his injuries and painful hospital experiences as many clinical studies suggest. Perhaps doll play might make it possible to explore these issues.

As I began to know Joel, my supervisor suggested that we bring his entire bed into the playroom. How his world opened up! On his first visit, I remember standing between two beds, Joel on one side and a 4-year-old boy on the other side. Just by placing a pillow at Joel's back, he could turn enough to see the array of playroom activities. I thought both children might enjoy running drumsticks along the railings of their beds. Very quickly our corner became the band with much clanging, clacking, and jingling to be heard. Although his partner laughed and sang, Joel made no verbal sounds while he played with the instruments.

We brought Joel's bed into the playroom each morning. When he had a partner, he liked to throw balls back and forth. Other times, he and I would make roads on a tray in his bed and he would move the cars and trucks about. I would make appropriate, or close approximations anyway, of traffic noises. Joel remained quiet.

As his mobility improved, I was able to put a wedge under his back and head so he could see and manipulate materials more easily. Play dough became a favorite. He worked hard at squeezing the different shapes and tearing them into small pieces, which of course were thrown all over the place.

I introduced some more banging materials, and Joel banged enthusiastically—over and over he banged. Eventually, I created a rhythm for his stick banging by clapping my hands and singing children's songs to his accompaniment.

Next he chose colored markers. While I held the paper, he drew lines all over. As he was on his back using his hands and arms for the first time in many weeks, his motions were jerky and stabbing. Even though he did not know how to use the pens, he smiled a great deal during the creation of his work. For several days he worked with the markers, yet although smiling and active, he remained completely quiet.

I noted how Joel hated having the adhesive bandage tape removed because it pulled on his skin. When applied, it was even worse in that it restricted the movement of his arms. I let Joel place tape on and then remove the tape from his restraints. He did this repeatedly.

Building on this play with the adhesive, I developed a medical play focus. As Joel was always in bed, materials had to be workable while lying down. Early in our relationship, I brought Joel a hospital doll. He often hugged it, and it seemed to provide him comfort. To encourage fine motor skills and expression of emotions and to increase his sensory experiences, I brought sheets of tissue paper for him to tear and crumple. I thought he might use the tissue to fashion restraints for his doll. Knowing that he might not want to do such an unpleasant thing to his loved doll, I gave him the choice. However, he seemed quite fascinated by the project and spent many minutes putting on and pulling off the paper restraints. I named what he was doing and reviewed why the restraints were necessary for the doll and reflected that the doll might not like them.

We continued to build on the theme of stickiness and increasing his fine motor skills. I gave Joel sticky contact paper with many little pieces of tissue paper to strengthen his fine motor activities. He loved the feel of the stickiness and spent much time putting his hands on it. Eventually he began to arrange the pieces of tissue paper and soon covered the entire piece of contact paper. He now had a growing art collection and developed a concept that stickiness can be pleasurable as well as painful.

I designed a cornmeal project. My plan was to use syringes for making designs with glue over which we would sprinkle corn meal. By now Joel could sit up at the craft table with a group of children, though tied into his wheelchair. Joel showed great fine motor control, squeezing the glue out of the syringe and sprinkling cornmeal over it. Quickly he found that sinking his hand into the cornmeal and squeezing it all over the table was much more appealing. This pleasure was exceeded only by swiping the cornmeal back and forth over and off the table. Such messy, large body movements are age appropriate but probably not in a hospital playroom. We decided that this was an activity best done outside. We also realized that it had been months since he had been outdoors.

I assessed Joel's readiness for play each day to determine if and at what level Joel could participate. Proceeding from his beginning involvement with adhesive tape, I decided to add other medical items, such as adhesive bandages, cotton balls, tongue depressors, and alcohol wipes.

He played with these simple medical materials for only a short time. I suggested we try using his doll, saying that we could see how the tubes and such could be placed on the doll's body to make it well. As Joel responded, I then added potentially more anxiety-producing items such as the large syringes used to suction out his gastric tubes, the smaller medication syringes, the gastric and IV tubing, an anesthesia mask, and the Broviac equipment. I gradually worked toward using the soft, realistic doctor and nurse puppets to allow Joel to act out medical interventions on his doll. My plan encompassed a wide range of activities as I knew Joel would be hospitalized for many weeks and we would have time to develop elaborate medical play.

The first step proceeded smoothly with Joel examining all the pieces I had gathered. He was fascinated by alcohol wipes, tearing open many of them. He would pull out the wipe, smell it, and wipe himself and things around him. He enjoyed sticking the adhesive bandages, so I extended this phase by assisting him in the creation of a collage. Joel was quite pleased with his creation and we hung it over his bed. It was the first time anything Joel had made was used to decorate his space.

The next phase in his medical play curriculum came after several days. When he seemed uninterested in what I brought him, I was ready to offer items more specific to his hospital experience. As he was still in bed, I brought in a hospital wash basin with a collection of the equipment I had seen used on him. He showed great excitement and some anxiety about several of the materials. He immediately took out one of the small syringes and began to pull the plunger in and out. He took the large syringe and placed it into a tube similar to his gastrointestinal tract (GT) drainage tube, and then he pulled back the plunger. He must have observed this procedure many, many times a day, and now it was his turn to do it. This play allowed him to handle the threatening equipment and gain a sense of control and mastery.

He was particularly anxious about the anesthesia mask and never chose it from the collection. When I lifted it out of the basin, he pulled back and gave a small cry. His surgery to insert his intestines into his body had occurred only weeks previously. Memories of the mask may have been too vivid. I gave it a name, briefly explained its use, and returned it to the basin. It was important to acknowledge for the moment that this item was too anxiety filled to be addressed. However, it would be important to return to the mask later so that Joel could work through his fears and gain a sense of mastery over this experience.

As before, Joel needed several days to explore the new collection of equipment. When his interest lagged, I suggested we try using his doll to see how the tubes and such could be placed on the doll's body to make it well.

Knowing that 2-year-olds have egocentric perceptions of the world, I felt it imperative for Joel to begin to understand he did not cause his injuries and he was not a "bad boy." Also it was important for him to know that he was not "bad" if he cried during the many different medical procedures he received.

Because of his age and regressed level of communication, we could only "talk" by using his doll as a substitute. I could talk with the doll about what was happening and tell the doll that it "was not a bad doll and that painful medical procedures were not a punishment." Joel's doll was very important to him. He carried it everywhere, holding it tightly when he endured unpleasant experiences.

Our work together was successful for a variety of reasons. Joel began to sit, reach, and manipulate items in his world. One day an 8-year-old girl joined our play. She had extensive hospital experience and wanted to put all the equipment on the doll in the correct places and loved to discuss the function of each piece. Joel appeared to enjoy her leadership, imitating her actions and laugh. Importantly, when she placed the anesthesia mask over the doll's face, Joel bent low over the doll to see clearly what was happening. He made the same movements himself. The three of us stayed in the playroom more than an hour repeating these activities. Although the playroom had been closed, the two children did not notice and kept manipulating the different items until a level of satisfaction and relief had been accomplished.

Each step of my project took longer than anticipated because of the unpredictability of Joel's schedule, his physical condition, and his need to work on the different stages of his play longer than I had planned. Currently we are using the nurse and doctor puppets to explore his feelings about their roles in relation to himself. I am considering enacting some dramas with him using the puppets. In the beginning of this dramatic play, we will encourage him to eat, an anxiety-laden situation for him. We have been working on encouraging the nursing staff to let him play with his food.

In that I was a student, I could not see Joel for the week of my spring vacation. On my return, I found Joel much better. The nurse was dressing him for the day in regular clothes free from any attached IV's. After inviting him to the playroom, I went on to talk with other patients. Soon I heard a commotion in the hallway and in moments Joel was walking into the playroom. He squealed with delight, and I jumped for joy myself! The morning was a celebration. We played ball, worked with play dough, and he climbed into a toy car and toured the floor hallways until we had to pry him out for a nap.

As Joel became more mobile, I observed his nurses becoming more affectionate with him. People went out of their way to visit his room, give him kisses, slap "high fives," or talk and play with him. It seemed that as his condition improved everyone was less fearful of making a connection with him. Hospital personnel have strong feelings about issues of child abuse. Further, when survival is in question, there is a tendency for all to keep a distance.

Joel's progress continued to be terrific. No more "Zip-Locs" stuck to his abdomen. He was testimony to the remarkable healing powers of the child. I hope that his emotional trauma can be healed as well. The entire staff has mobilized to help him. I explained to the staff the importance of allowing Joel to eat with his hands and permitting age-appropriate messiness. The staff was willing to allow the mealtime mess, even though more work for all was involved.

His physical therapy appointments provided great opportunities for me to share what I had observed about his behavior and preferences in the playroom and helped the staff encourage him to crawl and run about. We noted that he began babbling, and an occasional word entered his conversations.

Joel's second birthday approached. I planned to make cupcakes with him in the playroom. His aunt and uncle were to come on the weekend for a family celebration. Unfortunately, during the prior weekend, Joel spiked a temperature and clearly felt terrible. What a tragic setback. I spent his birthday morning beside his bed, holding his hand, rubbing his head, and just humming to him. When his nurse needed to take his temperature, I decided to assist her as I felt it was important to stay with him. I explained what was going to happen, helped roll him onto his side for the rectal thermometer, and talked softly to him throughout the procedure. (Usually the Child Life Specialist does not participate in medical procedures, but I felt he needed more support than his nurse was able to give.) He appeared to tolerate the procedure with only whimpers and small cries of protest. Afterward he calmed quickly, and we continued our time together.

Preparing for Discharge

The time was approaching for Joel's discharge. It seemed that each hospital department was making plans with little coordination. Early one morning his foster parents arrived to receive instructions about his physical care and to spend some time meeting him. They seemed sensitive, moving slowly toward Joel, until the mother was speaking to him as well as the other children sitting around the table. The foster parents followed us into his room and watched how I held him on my lap and which lullabies I sang as he went down for a nap. The foster mother wanted to hear about his favorite activities as well as what we do to personalize his care.

I decided to write a letter to Joel's new foster parents reviewing important issues:

> Joel will need help from his family to reinforce his strengths and support his efforts as he develops. The following is a summary of Child Life's observations of his likes and dislikes, as well as what behaviors fall within normal limits.
>
> In the hospital Joel has seen many faces each day, yet he has been able to differentiate by developing trusting relationships with the consistent figures. Trustworthiness will be reinforced if you always tell him what your plans are for him and what is about to happen. If it is time for a nap, explain why you are taking him to his bed and leaving him there. If you need to leave him with a sitter, explain you will be back. As he is used to many caregivers, he may not protest your departure in the beginning. However, once he accepts you as his special caregivers, you may see more complaints. When it's time for his medical procedures, explain exactly what you

need to do and how Joel can help you. Such behaviors will encourage Joel to believe what you say and trust that your actions are directly related to your care for him.

Joel has become used to the hospital as his home. Discharge will require time for him to master the new environment of your home. He may need extra comforting and, as most children, he enjoys snuggling. Other items that provide comfort are his train pillow and his hospital doll. He enjoys clutching these to his chest when he is tired or sad. He also uses the pillow to cover his eyes when he is tired and wants to sleep. If he is having difficulty going to sleep, it may help to rock him in your lap while you sing a quiet song.

We have noticed fine motor activities are a favorite of Joel's. He particularly loves drawing with markers or carefully making designs with glue. He will also love to sing songs with you and bang out rhythms with sticks or bells. He has helped us with cooking activities—carefully measuring, pouring, and mixing, and of course, eating. Joel will choose activities in which he can put small things into a larger container, particularly if it makes lots of noise! During quiet times, he enjoys listening to you read stories. He stays interested in storybooks and loves to look at the pictures.

We have been doing medical play with Joel, and you can continue this at home. Allowing him to manipulate the equipment you will be using for his treatments will make him feel less frightened during the procedures. Letting him practice with the equipment on his doll will give him some control over this part of his life. It is important for Joel to begin to master some of the fears he has about his many experiences in the hospital.

Joel's Discharge

Joel's past months of hospitalization have required much of him. He has met many people and they have come in and out of his life with few explanations and even less understanding by Joel. By providing Joel with frequent information, I have attempted to be a consistent caregiver, reliably appearing and disappearing. Now I must face the biggest separation—his discharge.

In a sense I prepared for Joel's discharge and my separation from him each day I was with him. As his discharge date approached, I talked about his leaving the hospital and his foster parents. At this point, Joel gave me no signs that he was listening—no head turned in my direction, no smiling or sad faces. No craft activities, no musical instrument play, and no fine motor activities for him right now. All he wanted to do was walk.

As I was able to be one on one with Joel, I spent entire play sessions cruising the hallways with him. Up and down the halls we went but never near his room. Possibly Joel worried I would put him back into his bed and he figured the best strategy was to stay far away from his room. Everyone wanted to say 'Hello" to Joel, but he would not stop. He was in control!

I prepared a portfolio for Joel to take home. His positive and negative memories of these months will be supported by mementos. Joel may also use the materials to talk about the unpleasant memories or at least have a vehicle to suppose what it might have been like. I included samples of his artwork over the months, cards he received, religious stickers that were over his bed, the poster I made for him describing favorite activities, and photographs of him and the various staff who had cared for him these past months. Perhaps these will stay a part of his life. At the very least, it will be something available if he wants to see it. It also made me feel better having something for him to take with him.

Joel's farewell party was held the day before his scheduled discharge. Leaving the hospital with his foster family will be enough excitement for one day. The day of his party began with the first real bath of his hospitalization. Although the nurses took in bath toys, he apparently screamed throughout the experience. Unfortunately, I was not included in the planning. From my Child Life knowledge, I would have introduced Joel slowly to water and bathing and given him more control. For him it was another unpleasant procedure.

Although farewell parties are not routine, Joel's was a combined birthday and good-bye event. Many people gathered—the nurses, occupational and physical therapists, speech therapist, surgeon, and Child Life staff, as well as other children and their parents. Joel never saw himself as the center of attention but seemed to enjoy sitting on my lap and tasting the soda and cake. Staff personnel needed to say their farewells. All worked perfectly as people posed with him for photographs for his scrapbook. Joel was willing to sit still while everyone came up to him and said their good-byes. Eventually, he chose to walk some more and the party broke up as the guest of honor strolled out the door!

Part Two

Child Life and Child Death

5

Harry

A 10-Year-Old's Last Summer

Lauren Manheimer

Harry, a bright-eyed, 10-year-old of African-American and Native-American descent, was hospitalized for a relapse of acute lymphocytic leukemia. At the time I met him he was confined to an isolation room because of the immunosuppressive drugs he was taking. Harry had been complaining to the nurses that he was bored. He was feeling relatively well and craved company.

The nurses, concerned about his isolation and boredom, referred him to Child Life. He became a priority because of his isolation, his dearth of visitors, and his medically vulnerable situation. I agreed to be his primary contact.

When I entered his room, he was lying in bed, channelsurfing. He welcomed me with a warm, teeth-baring smile. I introduced myself and explained how I might be able to provide him with a number of different activities that I thought he would enjoy. I reassured him that I was not a medical person but rather someone whom he could rely on to keep him company and relieve some of his boredom.

We soon found out that we were both afternoon talk show and MTV connoisseurs, and the ice was quickly broken. I suggested that we play a game and recommended several from which to choose. Harry selected Trouble. He seemed to enjoy instructing me in the way it was played.

We proceeded to play a tournament of the best out of five. In that the television was still on as we played, we jointly analyzed several music videos. When the television show discussed The Butterfly, Harry shyly showed me how to do this vogue dance. It requires a fair amount of rhythm to the hip-hop beat of a Snoop Doggy Dog song, and he grew enthusiastic about our dancing.

Harry had a good amount of energy and his spirits were high. I empathized that it was difficult to be cooped up in the hospital during the summertime. I let Harry know that I was committed to making his hospital experience the best it could possibly be. There was an immediate connection.

Harry had three siblings, and his parents had recently divorced. His mother quickly remarried a man from whom Harry felt estranged. He believed that his relationships with his younger sister, age 5, and his older sister, age 14, were exceptional. However, Harry explained that his eldest sister, age 17, was so involved with boyfriends, parties, and other teenage social activities that she had little interest in him. In that he worked for a traveling circus, Harry knew his father could not visit him in the hospital.

Harry expressed great admiration for his father, who was part Miwok and part Navajo. He spoke fondly of the pow-wows, bike rides, long swims, and fishing trips they had enjoyed together. Harry also believed that his father was a great and talented artist, and he proudly displayed many of his father's animal sketches on his hospital room wall.

Harry informed me that more than anything else in the world he wanted to be cured by his 11th birthday, the next month, so that he could have "a gigantic birthday party and invite all of my friends and family." He also told me that of all the colors in the rainbow he most loved blue.

It was the start of summer vacation, and Harry was remembering his favorite activities in which he could not participate because of his leukemia and hospitalization. He said it was unfair. He loved the summers with the circus, feeling the sun on his back, the salty taste of seawater on his skin, the sight of children playing in the sand, and the cool sensation of ice cream dripping down his chin. Most of all, he missed his long braids that had fallen out from chemotherapy. These comments came about when one day on looking in the mirror he remarked, "I miss my hair. I look funny." These topics were often prompted by what was on the television. Sometimes they came from exploring questions about favorite activities.

Harry carried an even larger burden. During his first bout with leukemia, approximately a year earlier, he developed a friendship with another hospitalized child his age who was experiencing a relapse. When this child died, Harry expressed deep concern for his own potential death. Harry had been consoled by friends, family, and medical staff that the other child died from a relapse, whereas he, Harry, was sick for the first time and would surely achieve lasting remission. However, with the onset of Harry's relapse, his deep-seated fears that he might not survive his illness were more threatening. Nevertheless he described his hopes, "I am going to be a tiger trainer when I grow up."

The next time I visited Harry in his isolation room I brought blue construction paper, magic markers, games, and a selection of books. Harry enjoyed art activities and especially appreciated my remembering his favorite color.

Over the next couple of weeks I worked with Harry at least an hour each day I was at the hospital. He knew when he could expect my visits. Each time we planned what we would do together. Together we read stories, wrote letters, played games, drew, painted, watched movies, listened to music, and danced to MTV.

On several occasions I tried to interest Harry in coming to the playroom to choose from a wider array of activities and interact with other children his age. He repeatedly told me that he did not want to leave his room.

I was concerned that Harry might be worried about how other children perceived him. After all, he was bald, attached to a number of IV lines, and needed to wear a mask if he left his sterile environment. His reaction was not inappropriate. Clearly, Harry did not look like an ordinary 10-year-old boy; however, in the hospital there were many children who looked like Harry, suffered similar illnesses, and felt as isolated and different from other children as he did. I believed that providing opportunities for Harry to interact with other hospitalized children would facilitate his mastery of anxieties and adaptation. Furthermore, an identification with a peer might foster a sense of belonging and mitigate his feelings of isolation, dependence, and passivity.

One particular afternoon I was able to convince Harry to let me introduce him to another 10-year-old, African-American, hairless oncology patient, Nate. In that Nate agreed to come to Harry's room, Harry could interact with another child without leaving the safety of his familiar room. The boys had much in common, played hours of Nintendo together, and developed the beginnings of a friendship.

Harry and Nate played together frequently during the next couple of days, and I was successful at convincing the two boys to join me in the Monopoly tournament in the playroom. Harry felt comfortable wearing a mask in public when he realized that Nate also was required to wear one. I, too, was willing to join the group of mask-wearers for the occasion. Harry told me later that he enjoyed the change of scenery and was looking forward to going to the playroom again.

Recalling Harry's love of animals and his desire to be a tiger trainer, I was overjoyed to learn that an actual trainer and a baby white tiger from Marine World were going to visit the hospital. The trainer was to appear on the patio that had both wheelchair access and electrical outlets for IV poles. Since Harry was in protective isolation and needed medication approximately every 30 minutes, I knew that it might be impossible to bring him to the patio. I was committed to making whatever accommodations and negotiations necessary to facilitate Harry's participation.

After an extensive amount of negotiation, the medical staff agreed to let Harry attend the outdoor event as long as he wore a mask and returned to his room for medication in precisely 25 minutes. Harry was ecstatic when I told him the news. I escorted Nate and Harry to the patio, the two boys giggling the entire way in anticipation. Harry took a seat in front so that he could pet the baby tiger and ask the trainer to tell him what it was like to work with animals. Although the 25 minutes went by quickly, it was a wonderful time. Harry now was absolutely certain that he would be a tiger trainer when he grew up.

Harry was able to leave the hospital and return home, but his physical condition rapidly became worse. On readmission, Harry was depressed and had severe pain in his chest and legs. He told me that he was angry with his mother for not visiting. She promised to come on several occasions, but she never came, offering only excuses. He was visited only by his 14-year-old sister. Harry felt lonely, isolated, and burdened with feelings of abandonment by his mother.

Since Harry abhorred the hospital food, he said that he was going to stop eating until his mother arrived with a home-cooked meal. With no sign of Harry's mother or home-cooked food, Harry began a hunger strike. I reported his predicament to the social worker, who promised to contact Harry's mother to encourage her to visit. In the meantime, I worked with Harry as often as I could to encourage his involvement in activities. I hoped he might use play to work through his painful feelings of passivity, abandonment, and victimization, and help him gain a sense of mastery and control.

Harry's mother came to the hospital relatively quickly after being contacted by the social worker. She brought with her a few of Harry's favorite movies and some home-cooked food, which he claimed was rotten. Perhaps Harry had envisioned that this food would be the best he had ever tasted, or maybe he had magical wishes that it would somehow make everything better. In any case, Harry definitely seemed more animated and less depressed after his mother's visit.

During her visit I noticed that Harry's mother was fidgety, repeatedly leaving his room throughout the day. Even when she was with Harry, she seemed elsewhere. I wondered how she was responding to her son's illness and the grave uncertainty surrounding his prognosis. Harry said, "My mom's being weird." She later explained she did not want him to see her crying.

After one month of Harry's hospitalization, I had the opportunity to attend oncology rounds. I learned that Harry was becoming extremely neutropenic with an invasive bodily fungus that was not responding to medical treatment. It was decided that Harry needed chemotherapy again, which meant at least another month of hospitalization, his third consecutive month.

Harry was being given a drug that caused him to sleep for most of the day. During his waking hours, he seemed more sad and withdrawn than before. Even though his desire to eat had significantly improved, he now had severe stomach pain and eating became an exceedingly difficult task.

The social worker felt that Harry's mother was extremely anxious about Harry's condition and denied his poor prognosis. She seemed to be shutting herself off from Harry in

an unconscious effort to protect herself from what was un-
bearable. Both the social worker and the psychologist
planned to meet with Harry's mother to offer her support
in dealing with her feelings and to emphasize that in this
time of crisis Harry was in desperate need of her warmth
and support.

A week passed in which Harry slept though most of each
day. On one particular afternoon, I found him awake. His
physical condition had deteriorated. He was thin and weak,
his skin yellow, and his speech labored. The whites of his
eyes had turned a blood red color from the fungus and there
were deep black rings below them. However, Harry's smile
of recognition welcomed me.

Lying alongside Harry in his bed was his father. I was
touched by his unabashed tenderness toward his son. He
gently stroked Harry's face and kissed him every so often on
the forehead as he spoke in a soothing voice. Harry's father
told him stories of his childhood and recited folktales of his
ancient Miwok and Navajo tribes. His father was pleased with
my interest in the stories and he proceeded to show me the
pictures of the ancestors that he had brought for Harry.
Harry seemed proud and peaceful. I believe his father was
able to provide him with reassurance and a sense of faith
that helped him endure the pain of his disease.

Not long after, Harry's condition worsened. He was
moved to Intensive Care. I was concerned that Harry might
believe that his illness was terminal and that he was placed
where he would soon die. I was concerned that being suddenly moved to a new room with unfamiliar nurses would
intensify his fears.

When I went to see Harry in the ICU, I was pleased to
find several family members by his side, looking at old photos
and telling stories. Harry's new room displayed all of the
same artwork that had once decorated his former room.
Although it was not the same space, it was personalized and
conveyed Harry's good spirit, his love of animals, and his

favorite color, blue. Harry never complained about his treatment, often reiterating what must have been told to him: in spite of the pain, the treatment was necessary.

Although Harry no longer had the strength to be involved in art activities or games, he enjoyed being read to, watching movies, and rapping along to MTV. Occasionally, he would ask me to draw something for him. He told me his creative vision and then directed me in marking the paper as he described. Meanwhile, Harry's father was intensely working on a drawing of an eagle that he planned to display proudly above Harry's bed.

Harry progressively worsened. His doctors decided to stop administering chemotherapy since his body was weak and the drugs were ineffective. Aside from trying some experimental treatments, there was now little more that medicine could do.

In private, Harry's father expressed to me his deep sadness that he was going to lose his only son. He verbalized how he wished that he had spent more time with Harry to show him "the way" of his culture. I reassured the father that from what Harry told me, he loved his father dearly and was very proud of his Native American heritage.

I was no longer able to draw with Harry since his speech had become so labored that it was nearly incomprehensible. However, Harry still smiled when I came in and enjoyed having me sit by his side, hold his hand, and read to him. Harry never spoke to me directly about his impending death. I believed that he was aware of it in his silence and felt as much peace as he did fear. Harry was a bright boy and probably surmised that he was going to die because he had known another child who had died under similar circumstances.

During one afternoon together, Harry began to cry and his father stood close to him and said, "My son, there is no need for tears. You remember what we spoke about." Harry's father handed his son his completed drawing of a soaring eagle. Harry held it against his chest, shut his eyes, and appeared tranquil.

I wondered what it was that they had spoken about. Did Harry know that his pain would end? Would he, in his death, become an eagle, freed from the shackles of his suffering? Was Harry to die quietly and with inordinate dignity? Did he believe in his heart that he was going to a better place, where his long braids would swing free, and he could join children in the sand with ice cream dripping down their chins?

Throughout the next week Harry's condition deteriorated and he could no longer breathe on his own. High doses of morphine kept him in a state of semiconsciousness. I continued to visit Harry to provide him with as much comfort and support as I could. Harry's family appreciated my dedication to their son.

Harry died 6 days before his 11th birthday. He was surrounded by his family members and the medical staff who had grown attached to him. Earlier that morning I had helped negotiate with the hospital's Security Department to grant his 5-year-old sister entrance to the hospital. She wanted to say good-bye to her brother. I felt that if she were unable to see him resting peacefully she may conjure up deleterious fantasies relative to his death. I stayed close to her throughout the difficult experience and answered her many questions fully in understandable language. She wanted to know what was happening, what was in the IV bag, why was Daddy crying, why was Harry so hot, is he sleeping, what is the nurse doing, is he dead yet, should she say good-bye, what should she say? Many of the questions had no answers. When I did not know the answer, I told her so.

For the last hour of his life, Harry was attached to what seemed like an endless collection of machines. Tubes entered and exited from various different places in his body. His skin was hot, swollen, and discolored. His eyes fluttered three-quarters closed. His tongue hung lifelessly between his teeth. Upon her request, I held the 5-year-old sister in my arms and brought her over to her brother. She gave him a kiss on his forehead and said softly, "Good-bye, Harry. I love you." The room was a sea of tears, both in sadness for the loss of a loved one and for relief at the end of Harry's suffering from a cancer so invasive that it stupefied even the most knowledgeable and skillful medical personnel.

Harry's arm began to twitch momentarily and his tongue danced between his teeth. His parents stood by his side holding his hands tightly, caressing his head gently. "We love you, Harry," they called out to him. "We are here for you. We believe in you. Your soul is beautiful . . . Go on, son. Fly away. Like an eagle, fly, fly away." The boy's mother was shaking uncontrollably. His father appeared calm. He tenderly placed a necklace around Harry's neck and burned sacred cedar incense. The pendant was made of feathers, which symbolized the eagle, his totem, and the power of flight. It was interlaced with beads representing his family's tribe and leaves of sage that held the powers of purification and benediction. The medical staff informed the family that Harry's tissues were dying and that only the respirator was sustaining his life. To turn it off would be to allow Harry peacefully to die. With the flick of a switch all of the lines on Harry's monitors smoothed into horizontals. Harry's father released a thunderous scream, and my stomach clenched and fell.

I received thanks and tender embraces from family members. The nurses removed the tubes and needles from Harry's lifeless body. They wiped away the blood that encircled his mouth, allowing Harry to rest peacefully with his sacred eagle feather on his chest. "You gave him life," his father told me. "Harry loved you."

I tried to remain collected but to battle against my tears seemed futile. I was bombarded by memories of Harry: our first game of Trouble, our Monopoly tournament, our trip outside to see the white tiger, our cooperative drawing, the singing and dancing to MTV videos, and, most of all, Harry's contagious smile. I had made a valuable connection with Harry. I had promoted his childhood and supported him with warmth and respect. He lighted up each time I came to see him and would inquire as to when I would return. I believe, in my heart, that even though I could not alleviate his physical suffering, I was a social stimulus and an emotional comfort.

Harry's funeral was the day after his 11th birthday, an event he had spoken of with great joy and anticipation. Not only did I feel that it was important to attend to show my support and respect for the family but also to provide myself with some emotional closure. Moreover, I felt that it was important to represent the hospital. After all, the staff had essentially been a surrogate family for Harry.

The ceremony was held in a Baptist church. Over 100 friends and family packed into the small church to mourn Harry's death and seek comfort in one another. Many prayers and songs were shared in Harry's memory to celebrate the freeing of his soul. The sermon was spirited and hopeful. The preacher declared to the congregation, "Don't cry tears for Harry, for he now dwells in a better place, basking in the sunshine of the Lord."

After the service, we were directed to the cemetery where Harry would be buried. Harry's Native-American relatives performed a Miwok–Navajo ceremony in which they burned sacred cedar and sage and gave offerings of food to the spirits who were guiding Harry to the other side. Drums were played as Harry's father explained the ritual and proceeded to bury his son. Immediately following the ceremony, Harry's father approached me and proclaimed, "You are his angel." With these touching words, I believe he was saying thanks.

I was deeply touched by the richness of Harry's culture. Working with Harry, I developed a keen appreciation for its customs that have enhanced my appreciation of cultural diversity.

My relationship with Harry was emotion filled, perhaps because it was my first close encounter with death. Although my feelings were strong and convoluted, I do believe that I sustained a professional ability to help Harry cope with his pain, fear, and loneliness. Nevertheless, at the moment of Harry's death, my professionalism and knowledge of the therapeutic relationship were temporarily annihilated. I felt a genuine loss and grief. I do not blame myself for surrendering to my feelings since my sensitivity, empathy, and humanitarian instincts are what drew me to such challenging work in the first place. Although having my heart invested in my work increases my vulnerability and emotional labor, it also provides me with rewards that constantly reinforce the importance of working with children in need.

A Note from Evelyn Oremland. It is from the notes on Harry that I initially developed the principles of the "play partnership" noted in chapter 1. On various levels, these principles characterize the play relationship in the situations described. It is because of, but not limited to, the loss of Harry that the essences of the play partnership became prominent.

Considering the emotional labor involved, it is important to realize that emotional labor is a category of work—the effort it takes to control one's own emotions in order to help others deal with theirs. Emotional labor is inherent in the role of Child Life. It can be argued that with less given there is less danger in terms of emotional labor. Yet with less given, one wonders if the Child Life role is adequately fulfilled.

In that emotional labor knows no territoriality—nursing, social work, medical-surgical, and Child Life—we must think of protections. Recognition of reality in terms of personal and time limits is important. We know that we cannot fill all of the needs of a child. The Child Life Specialist cannot *be* the parent who is missing.

To help the child deal with the situation adds focus to the work as well as recognition of the importance and the lack of importance that one has to the child and family. Further, ideally, the Child Life Specialist is provided with sufficient supervisory and consultative help with unusually difficult situations.

6

Dana

A 7-Year-Old Girl
with Leukemia

Jacqueline McCall

Dana, a 7-year-old Latina, was admitted for myelogenous leukemia. Our introduction came through my supervisor, "This is Dana. She can tell you everything about the hospital!" Dana was wearing a black-and-white checked dress with a shocking pink sash, a matching hat with a large pink flower, white tights, and black patent shoes. She wheeled her IV pole as though it were a fifth limb. I soon learned that Dana loved fashion, especially hats, which disguised her lack of hair.

Dana's Illness

Dana attended her first day of second grade even though she had not been feeling well. She saw her pediatrician after that first day, and the next day she was diagnosed with acute myelogenous leukemia. Dana was hospitalized immediately. She never returned to school.

A bright child with enormous sensitivity, Dana was also very sick. Until recently she had been a healthy child living a full and active life. Dana's cancer was a new concept for Dana and for her family.

She was hospitalized from September to April. During that time she went home for one week at Christmas. At a particularly difficult time during Dana's stay, her mother told me that what Dana needed more than anything else was to be home to "remember who she is." The mother was determined to make the doctors understand this idea.

On readmission it was obvious that Dana's time at home with her family had helped. She seemed lighter, dancing down the hall and singing. She spoke of the fun she and her family had had when visiting Santa Cruz. They stayed in a hotel, which she had never done before.

On the second morning of Dana's readmission, she was again sad. She confided that it was hard to be sick. I think the combination of the chemotherapy and her memory of hospital life quickly withered Dana's spirit.

There were only a few days that I did not see Dana up and about at the hospital. She attended hospital school and visited the playroom for activities. School at the hospital was a struggle for Dana, although the teacher noted she made progress. Games are often played as a way to teach the children. The hospital teacher told me that in the beginning Dana had difficulty socializing. She wanted to do everything first and not take turns. She was "not a good sport and was a quitter." The teacher attributed this attitude to a lack of discipline at home. Dana improved, however, and she learned to take turns. The teacher believed she needed the group experience.

Dana could not read. At times when I would read to her she would recognize a word, say it, and become frustrated that she could not read more. The hospital teacher recommended a tutor. He instructed Dana three times, but then he stopped coming to the hospital.

When Dana left the hospital in April in remission, her parents were struggling to decide whether Dana should undergo a bone marrow transplant. They decided that she should have the transplant in the hope that there might be a full recovery. No one in Dana's family had matching bone marrow, so Dana would have to harvest her own bone marrow while in remission. At one time, Dana's mother considered having a fifth child in the hope that that child's marrow would match Dana's. That this thought was seriously considered indicated the strength of the mother's desire to provide her daughter with what she critically needed.

Dana went home and the family prepared for the bone marrow transplant. Dana was happy when she came to the hospital for the marrow harvests. She danced and sang down the corridors, enthusiastically relating the fun she was having on family outings. She proudly showed that her hair had begun to grow. Life was becoming normal again, and Dana glowed with the pleasures of restored family life.

In June Dana's cancer relapsed. I know that the first relapse is the worst time in a child's illness. The family's best efforts have been thwarted. Compliance and hard work have been in vain. The patient and the family are forced to come to grips with reality and the threat of death. Dana's parents were devastated. The mother felt that Dana lost her chance for the transplant because the doctors waited in making the decision. She blamed herself for not being more aggressive. They held little hope Dana would go into remission a second time and she did not. Dana remained in the hospital until her death less than a year later.

A fungus due to the chemotherapy began to grow in her nose, and the doctors decided to discontinue chemotherapy. The parents were told that Dana probably would not survive. There was a marked change in the parents and in Dana.

They guarded their time with her, preferring to be alone with her. Dana, too, did not ask to see people as she previously had done. The family grieved what they were about to lose.

When the parents were not there, it was not unusual to find Dana in the corner of the playroom lying on the mat, silent and pensive. At these times she liked to have a Child Life Specialist or other volunteer with her offering a blanket, covering her up, and making her feel cozy. She did not engage in conversation, but she enjoyed the proximity of an adult and having her back stroked. I silently rubbed Dana's back many times. Dana was never shy about asking for what she needed, making comments such as, "Who can stay with me?" or, "Can you sit with me while I eat lunch?"

Her moods were as capricious as her illness. It was not unusual for Dana to be smiling and involved one moment and pouting and withdrawn the next. Although her moods were somewhat attributable to the multiple medications she was taking, they largely were due to a sense of unrelenting loss.

I did not see Dana participate in play other than Nintendo. Although her room was filled with stuffed animals and dolls, playing Nintendo was her favorite activity. It was not unusual to see Dana and several other children in one room playing video games together. Most often Dana played by herself.

Dana refused to eat. Her meal trays were frequently untouched. Staff coaxed Dana to eat but to no avail. Eating was one area in which Dana was able to exercise control, posing special problems for the nurses and the Child Life Specialists. Many times I sat with Dana to "picnic" or eat lunch. She drank her soft drink and on a good day ate carrot sticks. Even ice cream bars were unappealing.

One day Dana and Nancy, an 8-year-old girl, had their trays brought into the playroom for lunch. The other child, a new patient, ate her lunch immediately. Dana looked at each item on her tray and remarked, "I hate it." Dana told Nancy, "I remember when I first came to the hospital. I used to eat too." Dana had understandably grown tired of hospital food and was depressed.

Dana also asserted herself by refusing to take her medicine, not an uncommon problem with hospitalized children. One day, an entertainer came to the playroom. Everyone was having a wonderful time, singing and clapping hands. A nurse approached Dana with a tablet that she needed to take. Dana smiled and refused. The nurse, not wanting to interrupt and well aware of Dana's pattern, told Dana that she would be back when the entertainment was over. Dana, smiling, pronounced "No!" and sat on her pill.

As expected, the nurse returned after the show to make sure Dana had taken her tablet. It turned into a confrontation with everyone in the room watching Dana and the nurse. Dana seemed delighted with her audience, even though she knew that she would have to take her medicine eventually.

Dana's Family

Dana was an affectionate child who loved to be touched. She was able to reach out to adults, and adults responded to her. She was intelligent and able to make friends in the hospital. As a system, Dana's family was dynamic and powerful.

Dana was born in San Francisco. Her mother believed Dana was a special child, "One who wanted to born, to come through her." She remembered that Dana was born with her hands open, a meaningful sign to her mother. When Dana was 4 years old, her father, a Latino musician, wrote a song for her. In the song he expressed his love for her, told her she had the sensitivity of the angels, and assured her that nothing would harm her.

Dana was the second of four children. Her older sister, Helen was 9; Her brother, William, was 4; and her sister,

Dina, 2. Dana's father was from South America and darker complexioned than her American-born mother. He ran a small business. Dana was a beautiful combination of both her parents. Early snapshots revealed an animated, confident child with lovely long hair. In more recent photographs, Dana wore a whimsical hat to cover her hair loss. I never saw Dana without her hat.

The parents dearly missed the family as it had been. The mother said wistfully, "You should have seen Dana before she was sick. She loved to dance. She was always dancing." One day, the father brought a home video of the family. One scene showed Dana in the bathtub, which embarrassed her. She became angry with her father and began to cry. It was difficult for him to understand how she felt. He had brought the video to cheer her, not to embarrass her. I held Dana as we sat in a chair after the incident. The father kissed Dana good-bye, obviously feeling hurt and probably angry because of the scene Dana had made. Dana said, "You know how much I love you, Daddy. I want you all (family) to come back tonight. Okay?" The incident clearly exemplified the stresses of illness on family.

The family had other problems with the hospital. Early on, the parents expected to use the playroom and staff as day care for Dana's siblings. At times, the father behaved inappropriately toward female hospital staff, which I believe reflected his personality, cultural differences, and his struggle to cope with the difficult situation.

Yet, the family was fun, affectionate, and able to experience joy together. On one occasion, I walked into the playroom and the father was playing a tape of his Latin music. The mother was standing at the table, smiling and gently dancing. For a short time she seemed to have forgotten her anguish. Soon, the mother asked the father to sing for us. He sang about a beautiful little girl who had been truly blessed. Angels held her in their arms, shielding her from all harm. It was the song he had written for Dana when she was 4 years old. Both the mother and I had tears in our eyes as we listened.

The mother was assertive and aggressively attempted to work the system. She gathered information and made numerous lists of the pros and cons in Dana's medical treatment, documenting her care. She made lists telling the nurse how Dana was to be cared for and lists of hospitals where Dana could have a transplant. Dana's mother often posted a sign on her daughter's door to inform staff that Dana was sleeping or resting, usually after Dana had had a bout with nausea and vomiting and little sleep. Although the mother's attentiveness may have made Dana's care more difficult for the medical staff, it aided her in making informed decisions and not giving away complete control to the medical community.

On the parents' last visit to the hospital, the father had a lengthy discussion with the mother of another cancer patient. He said he realized that ultimately he and Dana's mother had no control over Dana's life and as parents they could only do what they believed to be best for her. He implied that what was happening to his family had a "greater significance" but that he could never understand why this horrible event had befallen them. In a telling statement, the father once said, "I used to think every day was a loss. Now I look at it differently. Every day with Dana is a gift."

The impending loss of Dana had profound effects on her three siblings. Not only did they experience the impending loss of their sister, they also experienced the marked loss of their parents' availability emotionally and physically as they focused on Dana's care.

The mother's anxiety and ambivalence regarding Dana and what her illness was doing to the other children was apparent. One time, when Dana's doctors were considering surgery on Dana's nose but questioning whether she would survive, the mother tearfully told me, "If Dana died, it would be over. We could go on with our lives and the other kids won't have to be raised in a hospital. But still, we've gone this far. Dana could have Christmas." She spoke emotionally of having "to desert" her babies. Many times the other children would telephone her while she was at the hospital and beg, "Mommy, come home, come home."

Perhaps Helen was the most affected. As the oldest child and closest to Dana, Helen experienced the most visible difficulties. They were playmates and friends, as well as sisters. It was not uncommon for them to exchange clothes at the hospital. They held lengthy telephone conversations.

The mother related the following story that illustrates the anxiety, guilt, and confusion Helen felt. The previous night, Helen had cried and cried as she tried to fall asleep. The two girls had argued that day and Helen was upset. She told her mother she was afraid Dana would die. She pleaded with her mother to tell Dana how sorry she was that they had been fighting a lot. She was sorry she told Dana that she did not love her anymore, and she was sorry she told her that she (Dana) did not look like Dana anymore. How distressful this fight must have been for both sisters!

William began to have enuresis. One time in the playroom, he lost control of his bladder. He showed no emotion, said nothing, and continued his play.

The effects on the youngest, Dina, were the most difficult to assess. Her mother's unavailability was certainly her key issue. Dina was happy at the hospital when she could be with Dana and the mother. At times, Dina would be playing with Dana and run to touch her mother. Otherwise, I did not observe unusual behavior in her play. I do remember though that when Dana's appearance changed dramatically because of the nose fungus, Dina became exceptionally quiet for a long time.

Unfortunately, financial concerns influenced decisions that should have been free of such considerations. During one of my last conversations with the parents, they struggled with what to do with Dana's body when she died. It was important to them that she be buried, but cremation was less expensive, and the mother decided to cremate Dana. Such difficult decisions have to be made at the most stressful times.

Rarely did visitors or friends come to relieve and support Dana and the family. No family lived in the area. The maternal grandmother, who lived on the East Coast, was herself diagnosed with cancer during Dana's illness. The father's family lived in South America. Dana had only one friend who visited her regularly accompanied by her mother.

Dana's Death

Shortly before Dana died, I spent time with her. Her IV line had been broken by an inexperienced nurse, and the mother was furious. For the mother, the accident indicated that the hospital staff had given up on Dana, whose condition was deteriorating. Dana was upset. Her hands hurt, and she was frightened. While the parents tried to resolve the medical problems, I stayed with Dana. She was glad not to be alone. I was glad to be with her.

Dana died on the weekend. The family had spent the day at the hospital. In the evening, the father had taken the children for dinner. The mother had remained with Dana. Dana died peacefully.

When the father returned, Dana was lying as always, and at first he did not comprehend that she had died in his absence. He then picked up his lifeless daughter, and holding her close, he danced around the room with her and sang softly to her. The parents stayed until early in the morning.

The mother did not intend to speak at Dana's memorial service, although she changed her mind because she wanted to tell everyone not to be afraid of death. She told of Dana's death. She told the assembled friends that Dana took two last breaths, and the mother felt her soul move upward. She said she heard Dana say, "I'm right here, Mommy." The mother said it was like giving birth again.

The mother said that now nothing would ever harm Dana again. She told the small gathering how angry she had been with them. "Where were you when I needed you?" she asked. She said, "Even Dana's godparents deserted us. I cannot look in the eye any who came only after the end of Dana's life." She told them that they, "came today only for yourselves." The mother was never one to hold back.

Dana and Child Life

The role Child Life played in Dana's hospitalization was complicated. Several Child Life staff told me that working with Dana's family was extraordinarily difficult because of their neediness. Also the parents were quick to be angry and "always could find something wrong" with the hospital and the hospital staff. The family expected a lot from the entire hospital.

The parents often intimated that the hospital staff only sought to earn money and had little personal involvement with patients. At times they resented that the Child Life staff returned to their own normal lives outside Dana and the hospital. As well, the parents seemed to resent the Child Life staff's relationship with Dana. The mother resented that Dana could be happy at the hospital and that "all these people could love Dana and that she loves them back." These problems illustrate the difficulties that often arise between Child Life Specialists and families when a child undergoes a long hospitalization.

Nevertheless Child Life Specialists were beneficial to Dana because of the environment they provided and because they were consistent, caring figures. Because of Child Life, the playroom was a safe haven.

Child Life attempted to provide Dana with play that allowed continuing opportunities for mastery and control.

Through play and art, Child Life Specialists are uniquely positioned to interpret a child's symbolic language and discover what a child cannot express in words. This position helps the parents and the siblings understand the patient and themselves. As advocates for children, Child Life Specialists can guard against withdrawing from relationships with difficult or dying children, a situation that often occurs with other hospital staff. For parents, Child Life provides much needed listening without judgment. Parents of dying children need to be able to reminisce and to articulate their grief, anger, and shattered hopes, and to discuss the painful decisions they need to make.

I saw and felt the importance of balance in the Child Life relationship. A playroom needs to have rules and limits. Without clear limits, Child Life can become an exhausting, depleting job. Child Life Specialists need to balance the time spent with patients and their families and their outside lives. Child Life Specialists cannot become parents to the patient or to siblings. They can nurture and support but cannot parent.

With Dana and her family, I saw how critical was the understanding of family dynamics. As difficult as the siblings were at times, they needed access to Dana, their parents, and the playroom. For them, a support group for siblings might have been beneficial. After Dana died, William received a quarter from a woman from the Make-A-Wish Foundation. He intentionally scratched the side of her car with the quarter. At home, Helen saved places for Dana to sit next to her and saved French fries for Dana to eat.

I saw the importance and necessity of an interdisciplinary team, each professional doing the work for which he or she is trained, and interacting to meet the needs of the family. I also learned the importance of self-reflection, particularly in a situation involving the death of a child. At times, I keenly felt the distress of the mother's struggle, perhaps because we are both mothers. This work is the "emotional labor" of the job. In a sense, one must learn to be comfortable with the uncomfortable.

On those occasions when the father struggled to find the meaning of Dana's life, he found comfort in the belief that Dana was not just their child, that Dana belonged to all of us, and that she came to teach. Dana was a beautiful child and a beautiful teacher. I shall miss her.

7

Brief Encounters

JANETTE TACATA

Cheri, Age 10

Cheri, a 10-year-old Mexican-American, was first diagnosed with Ewing's sarcoma when she was age 6. At that time her left leg was amputated and she was given a course of chemotherapy. The surgery and chemotherapy were considered successful, and Cheri remained disease-free until age 8, when a recurrence was found in her lung. According to her clinical chart, Cheri's long-term outlook was poor, even with repeated treatment.

Cheri's parents were divorced. Her mother had remarried. She had one sibling, Ishmael, age 14. According to Cheri, her mother and brother were constantly at her side. She called her mother "overprotective." In my observations, the mother was calm, aware of details concerning her daughter's care, asked questions, and was open to my interactions with Cheri. She was committed to being with Cheri in the hospital and to balancing Cheri's needs with her job and her son.

Cheri had been a good student and mature for her age. She was both verbal and engaging. On this admission, she was withdrawn, preferring to sleep and be alone. Yet, she was open about her dislike of the hospital and repeatedly stressed how much better she felt when she was home. She was able to ask her doctors questions about their decisions concerning her care, and she tried to negotiate as much time away from the hospital as possible.

Both Cheri and her brother shared an interest in heavy metal and alternative rock bands. She told me that one of her favorite groups was Nirvana. I said, "Sometimes people who are into heavy metal and alternative rock have intense feelings inside. You have to be going through a lot in order to understand Nirvana." She replied:

> They are so deep. Have you ever seen their video? It shows lots of things about death, like the crucifixion and stuff like that. It's about a guy who is thinking about killing himself and what it is like to die. You can tell he's really thought about dying. He had a lot of problems. Did you know their leader Kurt Cobain killed himself?

I was a bit uncomfortable with this conversation, wondering what it must sound like to Cheri's mother. Suicide and death are threatening to talk about. Would she think I was encouraging her daughter to look at the dark side of life? Although I was hesitant to continue, I thought that her interest in these songs must reflect her thoughts. After all, if a child begins to talk about death in doll play, we would not suppress it.

I asked Cheri if her comments about Nirvana and the video about death reflected her concern about someone who had contemplated death. She said emotionally, "Yeah!" I asked her if she thought Cobain had anything in his life besides problems. She replied, "His kid, his family. That's worth living for."

On my next visit, Cheri and I talked about a variety of talk shows and movies. She told me about a talk show she most remembered on how chickens are raised on poultry farms. She said, "If you look at how chickens are raised, they are surrounded by germs, pecking at their own poop, and the germs flourish on their skin and aren't removed, and people consume these deadly germs that can have an effect on the body and eventually cause death." She continued, "There was a show called *Untamed Heart* about a young man who had a baboon's heart transplanted into him as a child and that this heart gave him a strange character. He was special, but he died of heart failure. He left the person he loved most in grief."

Every story Cheri related involved death or illness. I told her that I thought she had interesting and insightful observations about movies, music, and talk shows and that they might be worth writing down. She said, "I want to make a real book, not just pieces of paper." She indicated that she was interested in writing poetry and songs, a book on likes and dislikes about the hospital, and writing about life. She asked if I could bring some fairy tales to read to her.

As I left, her mother said, "She talked with you the most she has talked to anyone in 2 weeks. She even sat up, something she has refused to do." I found myself looking forward to working with Cheri! She seemed to respond to me, and I wanted to respond to her.

Cheri and I worked together on a book that she titled *Feelings and Concerns*. Initially, she voiced her feelings about abandonment and expressed her great dislike of the hospital. Her complaints turned to fear of needles, her frustrations with her brother's "bugging her all the time," and her desire to go home. As she spoke I wrote down her thoughts, reading them back to her so that she could clarify her ideas.

It concerned me that her mother and brother were in the room and could overhear our conversations. I wondered if Cheri had enough privacy. I was also concerned for Ishmael, about whom Cheri said some honest but negative things. "I hate it that my brother is in my hospital room because he messes my bed and watches TV all day without letting me choose which show to watch. I wish he wasn't around," she said. Of course Ishmael heard this and looked very sad.

I could help Cheri arrange solutions to some of her complaints such as the TV problem with Ishmael. I encouraged her to talk with Ishmael about how she felt and that with a TV guide they could together plan what to watch. However, there were many things with which I could not help. She talked about her wish that she did not have to have chemo and how she hated being in the hospital. She cried as she expressed how she wished she did not have to be poked, have her hair fall out, and vomit all the time. Helplessly, all I could say was that these are tough situations to go through.

I knew that Cheri needed to express her complaints. On the next visit, I brought up her interest in writing and asked her if she wanted to dictate stories to me. For the next 3 days, Cheri told me the most incredible stories!

A fairy with a broken wing was being chased by a wolf. Luckily, she found a rock with a crack down its side just big enough for her to slip through. There the fairy waited until the wolf fell asleep. In the middle of the night, she gently tiptoed out of the crack in the rock. The wolf, who had a highly developed sense of smell, awoke and resumed chasing her. The little fairy was so afraid! She thought she was going to be eaten alive for sure. However, just ahead was a small shack, ugly and tattered. She reached the door and knocked with all her might. An ugly fairy man opened the door. The fairy begged the ugly fairy man to let her in. The ugly fairy man happened to be a powerful fairy wizard. He said, "I'll do better than that! I'll turn the wolf to stone." With a wave of his hand, he turned the wolf to stone and fixed the fairy's broken wing as well.

Then the ugly fairy wizard said, "You must now marry me and stay with me forever." After many days, the fairy could no longer bear living with the ugly fairy man. One day, she discovered in a book that fairy wizards have hearts of gold. The next day, she went to the ugly fairy wizard and ripped out his golden heart, sold it, and married a handsome fairy man.

Cheri's stories carried a common thread—being a victim of fate and gaining control over fate. Striking was the anger and aggression in the stories: ripping out hearts, trampling bad guys under giant feet, slapping ugly people, and terrible deaths. She would become intensely involved in the stories, sitting up and talking fast. I could barely keep up with her.

I knew that I would be leaving the hospital soon. I told Cheri, to which she had little response, even though once when I had missed 3 days she scolded me mildly. I noticed that during our last 2 days together, Cheri drew pictures for her book to accompany the stories but dictated little.

I felt much sadness about leaving, and we were both tearful at the good-bye. Cheri helped me realize how often dying children know they are dying and that we join them in a conspiracy of silence, keeping them from telling us their fears, and making them even more alone with something that we all fear.

I later learned that Cheri developed a recurrence with extensive metastases. Her family opted not to resume treatment, and I have lost contact with her.

Lisbeth, Age 8

Lisbeth, an 8-year-old Chinese-American with cancer, was according to her nurse an "emotional shambles." It was reported that without respite, Lisbeth moaned and cried. Unable to be comforted, she repeatedly asked for "mommy."

When I first met Lisbeth, the nursing staff was trying to
have her urinate for a test. She screamed, "No! I don't want
to! I want to go home! I want my Mom! You're hurting me!"
I tried to comfort her, reflecting her feelings, and acknowledging her discomfort. I seemed to make matters worse. Her
crying became louder. She struggled with the nurses to keep
from having to urinate. When they finally forced her onto
the toilet seat, she continued her refusal, and the nurses
became very strict with her. One said, "It doesn't matter
how long you sit there. We'll sit here all day until you pee!"
I could do nothing to comfort her during this standoff. I
left feeling discouraged. I consulted with a Child Life Specialist who suggested a different approach. "Just walk in and
suggest activities without talking about her situation. Make
it all seem normal," she said. I was not entirely sure what
she meant, but I walked into Lisbeth's room with paper and
a pencil and asked calmly if there were anything she wanted
me to write to give to her mother. It worked! Lisbeth was
distracted and focused on the letter.

She said repeatedly, "Get me out of here. I want to go
home." I wrote the message and asked, "What's home like?"
She told me about her dogs, her room, and her favorite
foods. I wrote down everything that she said. She regained
composure and engaged enthusiastically in this activity.
Soon after, she began writing her own ideas.

At one point, she talked about chemo, her fear of it, and
how she did not understand what it was or why she needed
it. A nurse zoomed in and took over our conversation. She
explained the chemo and its purpose drawing a parallel to
Tide detergent and Extra-Strength Tide. I felt disregarded.
When the nurse told Lisbeth she had to have chemo or die,
Lisbeth became visibly upset. I tried to comfort her, but the
nurse stampeded over me. Lisbeth curled up in a ball, whim-
pered, and went to sleep.

I was angry with the nurse and with myself because I did
not deal better with her. Although I am no expert in chemotherapy, I know that the nurse's approach was insensitive

and too factual and terrifying for an 8-year-old child. What a shame that I could not work more with Lisbeth. She needed support, explanation, and protection! I think I had a lesson in the limits of being a Child Life intern.

Part Three

Child Life and Adolescents

8

Child Life
on an Adolescent Unit

SUZANNE BERKES

Candy, Age 12

Sunday Evening

The most significant event tonight was an interaction I had with 12-year-old Candy who was newly diagnosed with diabetes. From her hospital chart, I learned that her mother and father were divorced and that she had a stepmother. Her parents had a history of drug abuse, and the father suspected that the mother continued to use drugs. Candy, her twin brother, and other siblings divided their time between their mother's and father's houses.

I was struck by how unstable Candy's mother looked. Her hair was disheveled. Her clothes were soiled and inappropriate for the weather. Her face reflected strife. Lines and scars made her look older. She spoke louder than necessary, laughed inappropriately, was unable to maintain eye contact, and her gait was unsteady. I suspected that she currently was using or recently had abused drugs. How could this mother deal with a chronically ill child, I wondered.

In contrast, Candy looked well integrated. Her clothes were appropriate; her skin smooth and fresh. She interacted easily with staff and peers. When she told us that at school her teachers all liked her, it was easy to see why. Unlike her mother, Candy looked at others directly and had a charming sense of humor. She seemed comfortable in the hospital. Never would I have matched mother and daughter.

Candy came to the Teen Lounge with her roommate Rose, an 11-year-old African-American girl whose hair was shaved back and who had extensive bandages on her head from surgery. Joining them was Candy's best friend Sarah, who was visiting. We decided to play Scrabble. Candy was concerned about other children's diagnoses. She asked me about several children in the room. I did not handle her questions as well as I would have liked. I told her that she would have to ask the children herself. I later realized in a supervisory session that it would have been better if I had told her that I was not free to discuss other children's conditions. I should have stressed the privacy issue, adding that I also would not talk about her condition with anyone.

Later, Candy asked Rose about her illness. I let this conversation continue until I sensed that Rose was not comfortable with Candy's questions. Rose began the conversation smiling, but she became more somber. Her neck muscles visibly flexed with Candy's questioning. I interceded by asking whose turn it was in the Scrabble game. I thought that if Rose wanted to talk about herself, she would return to the topic; if she were uncomfortable, she could use returning to the game as an inconspicuous way out. The conversation did return to the game, and Rose again became at ease.

During the course of the Scrabble game, the subject of bridges came up. Candy made a surprising comment saying that if she were on a bridge, she would probably jump from it. She said that her life was "a mess right now." I continued being supportive throughout the evening, yet I knew that I had to take this conversation to a supervisor as soon as possible. Obviously things were not right with Candy.

Monday Evening

In the Teen Lounge this evening several projects were going on simultaneously. Some of the patients, including Candy and Thomas, a 12-year-old boy with cystic fibrosis, chose to work with the button machine, to create individually designed pin-on buttons. Rose and Thurman, a 12-year-old African-American boy with sickle cell disease, busied themselves with painting wooden toy cars. Johnny, a 12-year-old Hispanic boy with a stab wound from a gang-related incident, played pool on his own. Candy looked tired and depressed.

I discussed with two Child Life Specialists my conversation with Candy about the bridge. They suggested I leave a note for the social worker and that I tell Candy that I had told the social worker about the conversation. This was an extremely difficult situation for me in that I felt I had betrayed Candy's trust. Further I was concerned that I would not be able to act appropriately if Candy reacted angrily. The conflict in me was nearly overwhelming. It took me a while to integrate what I needed to do.

I talked privately with Candy in the Teen Lounge. I told her that I was concerned about what she had said about the bridge and I had felt responsible for discussing it with the social worker. I told her that the social worker would be talking to her about what she said. She seemed almost grateful.

Candy was concerned that she would not see me again before she left the hospital. She said that tomorrow, a day that I am not usually at the hospital, she wanted to take pictures of all the people who had been "so nice" to her. Clearly she had mixed feelings about leaving the hospital. I told her that I would drop by after my classes.

I visited Candy that evening for the picture. She introduced me to some friends as her favorite person in the hospital and took me to the cafeteria to introduce me to her father and stepmother. When she introduced me again as her favorite person, I indicated that Candy had met a lot of nice people at the hospital during her stay.

It would seem that my telling Candy that I would talk to the social worker about her suicide thoughts had solidified our relationship. I think she was relieved that someone took her seriously.

Manuel, Age 12

Thursday Evening

Tonight I met 12-year-old Manuel, who has lymphohistocytic erthrophagocytosis, a rare bone marrow disease. His eyes were notable—big, bright, and expressive. His smile rivalled his eyes in expressiveness.

Manuel was born in Mexico. His family came to the United States when he was 6 years old. His mother spoke only Spanish; his father spoke limited English. Manuel said that his mom was always around but that his dad usually was not because he had to work and they lived far away. Manuel was the youngest of five children and was especially close to his brother, Jimmy. The other siblings were girls.

Manuel seemed a little hesitant to join the group activity in the Teen Lounge. Both Johnny and Candy were experienced participants. Their familiarity with the environment made entry harder for the newcomer. Manuel played pool with Johnny, who was not interested in going easy on the new guy.

Terrance, a 13-year-old African-American with diabetes mellitis, came in with his family, who almost took over the Teen Lounge. The room was abuzz with pool, Connect 4, TV, and Ping-Pong. I felt a little out of control. Manuel left early when the scene became intimidating. I asked Terrance's siblings and mother to leave. In retrospect, I should have told Terrance's mother that all of her children could not be in the room at the same time.

Afterward, I went to Manuel's room to spend some time with him. I brought cards, and we played three games. We talked about "how crazy the Teen Lounge had got." I told him that the lounge would be open again on Sunday. I did not want Manuel to think that his needs were less important than anyone else's. He did not express any complaints, being a polite and undemanding person.

Sunday Evening

When the Teen Lounge opened this evening, Manuel headed straight for the pool table. Two other boys, visitors, began playing pool with Manuel. A football game was on TV.

Manuel mentioned that his brother Jimmy might visit this weekend. Sam, one of the visiting boys, asked Manuel why Jimmy was not here now. Manuel explained that his family lived far away. Sam was curious and amazed as to why Manuel came from a great distance to this hospital. At this point, I said that children came from all over to this hospital. Sam then asked Manuel why he could not go to his local hospital. Manuel said that this hospital was better at helping him with his disease. Manuel said, "If I did not come here, I would die."

Manuel then described his experience in the ICU last spring when he was extremely ill. He said he was connected to 12 IV's. When I looked a little surprised, he said that he had a Broviac with several lines attached to it. He was smiling and even laughing as he talked about this episode.

Manuel's casual and good-humored account of his experience in the ICU reflected some degree of mastery, although I was concerned about his complete even-temperedness in all situations. Even when losing games, Manuel expressed no disappointment or anger. I think it might help if he could express his emotions more, perhaps with clay or something he could punch.

Monday Evening

My supervisor started a game of Monopoly between Manuel and Woodrow, a 15-year-old boy with a severe skin infection who appeared developmentally delayed. I initially thought these boys were a poor match, that Manuel was much sharper than Woodrow. I was astonished to discover that Manuel could not add a simple sum of the two dice. At one point, he threw a "5" and a "6" and asked Woodrow what the sum was. My supervisor and I alerted the hospital school about Manuel.

He and I talked about his Spanish. Manuel said that he did not speak Spanish very well any more. No one seemed to know the true extent of his English. His reading and math skills seemed that of a third grader.

Wednesday Evening

In a conversation, it became clear that Manuel knew very little about his illness and how it was affecting his body. My supervisor and I discussed ways to help Manuel become more familiar with and gain understanding about his illness. We copied pertinent parts of Lynn S. Baker's book entitled

You and Leukemia. We discussed the pages we selected with Manuel's nurse and checked with the hospital schoolteacher to see if reading this book could count as a school activity.

I was not sure that Manuel would be open to such a project, however I was excited about providing him with an opportunity for learning. He is a special guy!

Sunday Evening

Manuel announced that he was going home that day. His father was there. I was sad thinking that I would not be able to develop the book with him. I was surprised at my conflicted emotions. I felt sad that he was going home! Of course he was happy about leaving the hospital after more than 2 weeks. He played pool in the Teen Lounge with a vengeance to the point where the pool balls were flying off the table.

Later I learned that Manuel was going to the Family House where families who live at some distance can stay when doctors want to observe a patient longer. If he were fever-free for several days, he could go home. When it came time to say good-bye, I was again conflicted. My inclination was to give him a hug, yet I knew that would be appropriate only if he initiated it. He looked at me as if he might want to hug me but midstream stuck out his hand for a handshake. I shook his hand and patted him on the shoulder. He smiled and said he would be by tomorrow for the afternoon Teen Lounge activity.

It was not yet really a good-bye. There was still the possibility of developing the book. I was struck by feeling sad and happy at the same time.

Monday Evening

Today was an incredible day in the Teen Lounge. I spent some time with Gary, a 15-year-old African-American with acute lymphocytic leukemia. We created a button-making frenzy with our great button-making machine. He made buttons for all of the nurses.

Manuel came from the Family House, and he and Gary had a pool marathon. My supervisor brought in a preparation-for-surgery book, which was a compilation of photographs showing the various people and places someone might sequentially see on the way to a surgery. Manuel and Gary were both interested in the book. Manuel was again getting a Broviac and Gary, a mediport. The boys swapped stories about their past surgeries, talked about preparing for surgery, the extreme tiredness they felt right afterward, and Gary talked about how "high" he felt on anesthesia. I asked questions to clarify their experiences.

At one point, Gary mentioned that both of his parents always came when he had a procedure. Manuel said that his mom usually attended but that his dad usually could not be there because he had to work and they lived far away. Gary reemphasized that his parents *always* came. I said, "Sometimes parents cannot be here even though they want to."

In describing his experiences, Manuel lifted his shirt to show us his scars. He had a Broviac and had had his spleen removed. I was amazed to hear all that these boys had to say to each other.

When Gary left the Teen Lounge, Manuel sat down with the leukemia book. At one point, he started talking about painful procedures and the difference between lumbar puncture and a bone marrow biopsy. He was graphic about the sucking up of the tissue in the bone marrow procedure. Using his hands, Manuel showed how he thought they twisted and pulled the needle. He said, "They pull and pull." He repeated his description several times. I asked him how he got through these painful procedures. He said he just held still. I asked him if he ever had anybody come with him when he had a procedure. He said that his brother came once, but his parents did not come. I must have looked surprised, because he added, "My parents don't come because the procedure hurts them more than it hurts me." I was moved by the maturity of his comment. I replied, "I understand what you mean."

Wednesday Evening

Manuel announced that he would be going home on Thursday or on Friday. I asked him what we should do about the leukemia book, and he said that we could still work on it together when he came to the clinic for his chemo.

Knowing that Manuel was about to go home, I asked him what he would be doing when he got there. He hesitated, "The first thing I want to do is to go to church." I did not ask for any clarification. He talked about his sister's getting married. I asked when the wedding would be and he said that it would be in a year. He also said that the wedding would take place in Mexico and that he could not go because he would have to wear a mask and the air was heavily polluted. He also said, "What would I do if I got a fever? Where would I go?" He seemed overly accepting of his condition—no hint of complaint, only a statement of fact.

During his hospital stay, he always accepted his situation and worked within the system. He was cooperative with the nurses and during treatments, used the resources available to him (the Teen Lounge, and so on), and was respectful of the constraints imposed on him. He never complained about the Teen Lounge having to close at a certain time or about people having to leave when they did.

A couple of times Gary wanted to take the pool table up to the fifth floor after the Teen Lounge was scheduled to close. Gary was not accepting of my not allowing the move. Both times, Manuel stepped into the conversation saying that the pool table stayed in the Teen Lounge and that it would be available the next time the Teen Lounge opened.

He added, "If the Teen Lounge was on the fifth floor, then maybe we could play with it longer . . . but it isn't. It's on the fourth floor, and so that's just the way it is." Gary accepted it a lot better from Manuel than from me.

Manuel and I also discussed his stay at another hospital. I asked him to tell me about it and if it were different. He talked about differences in size between the school and playrooms and mentioned that the other hospital did not have a separate Teen Lounge. He also said that the visiting age, unlike here, was 18 years, but that the hospital made an exception for his brother, Jimmy, who stayed in his room while Manuel was in isolation, which lasted over a month. He talked about what Jimmy and he did together. They watched movies, and Manuel mentioned that Jimmy drew a lot. He said, "You see, Jimmy worries about me, so he draws."

Thursday Evening

Manuel was to go home this evening and I found it difficult to say good-bye. When I arrived at the hospital I found my Child Life Supervisor in the Lounge with a teenager. She asked me to guess who was sitting with her. I instantly realized that it was Jimmy, Manuel's brother. My supervisor suggested that I say good-bye to Manuel.

I had a few minutes with Jimmy and Manuel, who was happy to be going home. They introduced me to one of their sisters, saying that she was the one who would donate bone marrow to Manuel at another hospital. Manuel explained that he would be hospitalized for at least a month for his bone marrow transplant. I asked him how he felt about that. He responded, "If they didn't do it now, I will just get sicker and sicker and sicker." I asked if he wanted to take the leukemia book with him. He said that I should keep it because he would forget it.

It is interesting to note that Manuel's mother stayed with him throughout his entire hospitalization. At night, she slept at the Family House. Each day she remained at his bedside, although she had no problem letting him leave his room to go to the Teen Lounge or elsewhere. I wonder how much Manuel's relationship with his mother has to do with his apparently mature ability to adjust to these trying circumstances. It would seem that she provided a basis for development of security within the hospital setting and all its many players.

Mary, Age 15

Monday Evening

Mary, a 15-year-old African-American, was admitted to "rule out" pelvic inflammatory disease (PID). Her 21-year-old boyfriend, I had heard, was HIV positive.

Mary is outspoken, yet cooperative. She and I spent a great deal of time talking about her boyfriend, whom she described as "quite a gentleman." She said that her parents initially were angry about the idea of marriage but that they have come to like him. I asked her how long they had been dating. She responded, "Four months, the longest I dated anybody." While we talked, she painted a wooden squirrel and made a banner for him.

Mary said that she felt more popular in the hospital than she was at school. I asked her to explain. She said that she talked to more people here and that more people knew her. She did not know why the two situations were different. I reminded her that she told me that she behaved differently in the two places. She agreed. She said that in general people were much nicer in the hospital. I was not sure how to respond.

Mary indirectly said something about feeling like a child even though she was a teenager. I confirmed with her that she was but 15 years old. She said, "Yeah, and here I am wearing a diaper." I did not know if she were making this up or if it had to do with her treatment. I later learned that she was wearing a diaper of sorts. I wished I had known about the diaper. If so, I might have said, "Sometimes the treatments you have to go through as a patient make you feel like you're a child. It's hard to remember when you're going through it that eventually they make you better."

Another adolescent entered the Teen Lounge. He painted a wooden car and was pretty quiet. I worked alongside both of them in silence. Sometimes I find the silences hard to deal with. I respect the child's right not to talk, but I also want an atmosphere of openness. I know that silences are a part of our work, but when I sit in silence with children, I wonder when is the right time to intervene. I know and can feel that a lot goes on in silence. The children are building trust in me and seeing that I am respectful of them. I often wonder if I am just sitting there and not talking because I want the children to take the lead. For me it is difficult to tell if it's the right silence at the right time. I will have to understand silences more fully to mature as a Child Life Specialist.

Thursday Evening

Tonight was possibly the most difficult night I have had at the hospital this semester. I left my coat in the empty Teen Lounge for a few minutes instead of locking it in the office. When I returned, my coat was gone. I asked a nurse if she had seen my green coat. The nurse became serious and said, "Ask Mary."

She started walking with me toward Mary's room. I indicated to her that I wanted to talk to Mary alone. Although Mary and I had not spent much time together, I felt that we had the beginning of a relationship. To preserve that relationship, I wanted to give Mary an opportunity to save face.

Mary was on her way home. I found her in her room wearing my coat. "That looks like my coat, which I left in the Teen Lounge a little while ago," I said. She responded saying that the coat was hers and that she had lost it on entering the hospital. Not wanting to accuse her of lying, I asked if there were gloves in the pocket. She said, "No." I asked her where she found the coat. She said that it was in the Teen Lounge. I said that if that were the case, it was my coat because I had left it there a little while ago. She continued to insist that it was the coat she had lost.

Without becoming angry or accusatory, I insisted that the coat was mine. Finally, she asked me if I wanted it, and she gave it back to me. She left rather cheerfully and told me to have a nice evening. The encounter never became angry.

What a strange position to be in. I wanted to remain true to my Child Life role *and* I wanted my coat back. Most of all, I wanted to avoid having the security guard intervene.

I knew that Mary was poor and did not have a coat to wear on this very cold evening. She probably did not know that the coat that she found was mine. I was naive to leave the coat unattended. Many of the children in this hospital are poor, and the temptation to take something that is not theirs is great. In the future I will act more carefully by helping the children avoid temptation and locking my things out of sight. I was really shaken and found myself hoping for a relatively easy and uncontroversial rest of the evening.

Abigail, Age 14

Monday Evening

We had a lot of fun in the Teen Lounge today. Abigail, a 14-year-old whose medical condition I did not know, Jorge, a 14-year-old with a scalp burn, Shawna, a 14-year-old with "rule out" appendicitis, and I played poker. Abigail came alive during this activity and led the group. Her laugh was contagious, and she was enjoying herself, a far cry from her first day in the Teen Lounge when she lashed out at everyone.

Abigail mentioned the coat incident several times, having been Mary's roommate at the time. Abigail felt that Mary wanted a lot of attention from everyone. Abigail had strong feelings about how she would have handled the situation. She said that if Mary had taken her coat, she would have yelled at Mary and demanded that she give back the coat. She said that I was much nicer and calmer than she would have been, mocking the way I spoke to Mary, but not in a negative way.

I learned that Abigail had been convicted several times for assault and burglary. She was currently serving her parole in a group home. At one point Abigail started to tell me about her "old life," as she called it, but another teen walked in and she grew silent.

Wednesday Evening

Abigail entered the Teen Lounge for a final visit and drew several pictures. First, she drew a picture of me saying that I was goofy, a sentiment she repeated frequently.

She was in good spirits about leaving the hospital and returning to her group home. She gave me a hug good-bye and again said that I was the goofiest person she knew. I was never sure what she meant.

9

*Preadolescents
in the Hospital*

JACQUELINE McCALL

Amanda, Age 9

Amanda was diagnosed with kidney disease at age 4. Now a 9-year-old, she had recently undergone a kidney transplant and had returned to the hospital because of seizures. When I first met Amanda, she showed me pictures of her family, home, new puppy, and boyfriend. She told me how she came to the hospital in a helicopter but had been too sick at the time to remember the ride.

In the playroom, Amanda sat with Dana, another preadolescent, and ate her lunch. I could overhear their conversation. They discussed Byron, a patient whom Amanda had not yet met. Dana told Amanda how handsome Byron was. Byron entered, and Dana, visibly happy to see him, introduced him to Amanda. Soon Byron and Dana moved to the Nintendo machine to play together and left Amanda alone.

I brought my lunch over to where Amanda was sitting and asked if I might eat with her. Amanda stared at Byron and Dana as they played their game and said, "That Dana. She's just making a fool of herself." I asked her why. "Because she has a crush on Byron," she said. I asked her if she had ever had a crush. She told me that she had made a fool of herself with her first boyfriend and she was not going to let it happen again. (Her comment seemed unusually adult.) I asked Amanda how she felt being back in the hospital. She told me the hardest part was seeing everyone sick. "I worry that it's going to happen to me. The doctors tell me that it won't, but they don't know. They don't know for sure." I told her I understood why she was worried. I also told her the doctors had lots of experience and were taking good care of her. I left Amanda after this conversation and moved to another table.

Soon Amanda moved next to me. She crossed her arms in front of her and watched Byron and Dana. She made faces and muttered quietly, "Oh, look at Dana go. Look at her make a fool of herself. She won't leave him alone." I suggested she sounded a little angry and asked if it bothered her that Dana left her alone and went off with Byron. She said it had. I asked her if she could talk with Dana about how she was feeling. She said she didn't want to. She wished someone else could tell Dana. I told her that I thought it would be best if she could speak to Dana but that I could sit with her and help her. After awhile she said she wanted to talk with Dana while I was there but without Byron.

I could tell that it was hard for Amanda to wait. She asked me several times when Byron was going to leave, heaving heavy sighs. Finally Byron left. Amanda signaled me to ask Dana to come speak with Amanda, which I did. Their conversation follows:

Amanda: "You know how you went off with Byron and left me alone?"

Dana: "I know, you're jealous just like I was when you and Heather were playing without me last week."

Amanda: "Not jealous exactly. It's more like not treating two friends equal."

(I wondered why Amanda needed me. These girls seemed more competent at expressing their feelings than many adults.)

Dana: "You said it was okay for me and Byron to play, and you didn't want to play with us."

(I suggested to Amanda that perhaps she did not say what she really meant.)

Amanda: "No, I didn't."

Dana: "I know what you mean. Sometimes I don't say what I mean either. Like when I'm afraid I'm going to hurt somebody's feelings."

Amanda: "Yeah. In my family everyone says no when they really mean yes."

Amanda: "I really don't want to get to know Byron because I am leaving the hospital on Friday and there's no point. And you're lucky, Dana, you don't have hair." (Amanda's aunt had earlier washed and combed her long, thick hair and it had hurt her.)

Dana: "Lucky? I'm not lucky. I want to have hair. But I see what you mean. Maybe you have too much hair."

Amanda: "Yeah, and I have hair on my lip and face (she brushes her finger across her upper lip). I have lots of hair on my arms and legs. I look different. It is the steroids."

Dana: "I look different now too."

I told the girls what a great job they did in talking together. Amanda said, "I wanted you here because I was afraid Dana would get mad."

10

Angel

A Failed Case

STEPHANIE ERNST

Angel, a white teenager, was admitted because of a septic knee resulting from improper care of a knee wound. She admitted herself and told the staff that she was 16 years old and had been dropped off by her foster mother, who gave her $20 and told her never to return home. Later Angel revealed that she lived on the streets as a prostitute. Past medical records indicated that she was 14 years old.

Of average height and with rather small features, Angel had shaved her head to about a half-inch except for one very long lock in front. She spent much of her time looking in the mirror examining this lock of hair, braiding and re-braiding it. Frequently, she would "fix herself up" and wheel herself to visit male patients.

113

Angel had a psychiatric history and was known to have spent a short time in a local county mental facility for observation and treatment. From admission, Angel displayed many behavioral problems. She would yell obscenities, assault staff members during procedures, and smoked in her room, which was strictly forbidden.

Angel's knee infection required an extensive intravenous antibiotic regime. The antibiotics were not working partly because Angel refused to keep her IV in place for the long hours that the treatment required. Eventually it was decided that she needed surgery on her knee.

Child Life and Angel

Angel was referred to Child Life by several nurses who were having difficulty dealing with her. When I entered her room, Angel was sitting in bed and greeted me with skepticism. I explained who I was and my role at the hospital. She seemed relieved that I was not there to discuss her medical condition or to perform any procedures. I offered her several choices of activities, which she declined. She chose instead to tell me her life story, focusing primarily on her boyfriend. I knew my role was to listen. We talked for about 20 minutes, and I told her that I would return for more conversation in 2 days.

The next day, Angel verbally abused the nurses and pulled out her IV. She asked to speak with me and was reminded that I would be in tomorrow.

When I returned to the hospital, Angel seemed glad to see me. She spoke very rapidly, as if she had a lot to tell me. She spent 15 minutes telling me how awful she had been to the doctors and nurses and how she "hated this hellhole." At times she sounded proud of her behavior and asked for my approval. I listened carefully, refraining from judgment. I was attempting to develop a relationship with her.

It seemed clear that she fantasized that the doctors and nurses were there to harm her. She seemed unable to understand that the medical interventions were to help her. Slowly I interjected some thoughts. I explained in basic terms that the medical team was there to help her so that she could leave the hospital. I told her that it was okay to cry and scream during painful procedures so long as it did not interfere with the treatment. She responded, "I'll try and go easy on the doctor next time." We discussed the IV "start" and ways to alleviate some of the fear and pain, such as looking away, squeezing a hand, and yelling. By coincidence, a nurse came in to start an IV. Although Angel cried and screamed, she cooperated fully, and the "start" was successful.

That afternoon I took Angel in a wheelchair to the outside courtyard for fresh air and a place where she could smoke. We talked about her hospitalization and the recent procedure. We talked about activities, and she decided that she would like to string some beads for a necklace. She was interested in making jewelry for herself and her boyfriend. We returned to her room and I sat with her for about 15 minutes while she put together a necklace. I told her that I would have to leave soon. After a few minutes, she pushed the beads aside and said that she wanted to lie down. I helped her out of the wheelchair and into bed. I told her I had to leave, and I said good-bye. She did not answer. When I was halfway out the door, she yelled, "Good-bye! I'll see you tomorrow!"

Before my arrival the next day, a doctor informed Angel that she would have to have surgery on her knee later that afternoon. She became agitated and aggressive. She screamed obscenities at the anesthesiologist and injured the anesthesiologist's finger. I was on medical rounds with the staff when Angel's nurse rushed up to tell us that Angel had pulled out her IV and was packing her bags to leave. I went straight to her room and found her frantically packing. I said, "You look angry. I see you're packing your things. It's hard to be here." I suggested that she stop for a minute so that we could talk. She was angry but not violent. She told me that she hated being in the hospital and was not going to let anyone "cut up her knee."

At that point the doctor came in. She began to threaten him, "If you come near me, I'm going to hurt you!" The doctor replied, "Go ahead and hit me. I don't care. You know I like to fight." She turned around and began to hit him. He did not stop her. She tried to run past him, but he grabbed her around the waist. She then tried to bite him. He replied, "Go ahead and bite me. It won't hurt." He encouraged her to fight, and her anger and aggression increased. She clearly lost control.

I was somewhat concerned for my safety and felt that there was little I could do. I decided to leave and began helping disperse the crowd that had gathered and calming the children in the neighboring rooms. Hospital security arrived. The guards restrained Angel, and she was given a sedative. Later that day, Angel had her surgery, and she remained restrained in her bed over the weekend.

On Sunday, Angel convinced the nurses to remove her restraints. Later she locked herself in the bathroom and threatened suicide. She was placed on 24-hour watch and was heavily sedated.

Monday morning I went to see Angel. She was still heavily sedated. She managed to say hello. I invited her to join us in the playroom later in the day for some music.

I went to see Angel again after lunch. She was sitting in her wheelchair. She greeted me with a hug. She was clearly more coherent than she had been that morning. We talked about the weekend, but she had little to say. I invited her to the playroom to listen to some folk music. I wheeled her there, and we sat together and listened. The next day, Angel was in better spirits. She requested some materials for coloring and spent the day engaged in this activity.

The following day, Angel greeted me with a hug and talked nonstop about how she was going to be discharged later in the day. Neither she nor I knew that she was to be discharged to the county mental facility where she had previously been a patient.

While I was with another patient, the social worker and psychiatrist told Angel that she was to be discharged to the facility. Everyone could hear her screaming throughout the ward. Security was called. Then everything became quiet. About 10 minutes later, the psychiatrist came and told me that Angel had asked to see me. The psychiatrist told me that initially Angel was angry and agitated. She was offered sedation but refused it. She crawled into bed and said that she wanted to see me "but did not want to get angry and hit me."

I felt nervous on entering the room. Although I knew she had the potential to become violent, I was never afraid she would harm me. I was more concerned about what I was going to say. The psychiatrist stayed at the door. I went into the room and found Angel in a fetal position in bed. She was under the covers and crying softly. I sat down next to the bed and rested my elbows on the edge so that I could be physically close to her. Our conversation follows:

Child Life Student: "I hear you're having a rough day."
Angel: "Yeah. I have to go to the f——g hospital again!"
Child Life Student: "What hospital is that?"
Angel: "It's a f——g mental hospital! I've been there before and they lock you up and you can't do nothing."
Child Life Student: "I wonder why they lock you up."
Angel: "I don't know—to tick you off!" (She laughs.)
Child Life Student: "It sounds like they want you to be safe. I think this is what this is all about. Doctor . . . "
Angel: "Don't say that b——d's name!"
Child Life Student: "Okay. The doctors and nurses and I all want you to be safe. That's why we are having you spend some time there. It sounds like you're worried about being locked up."
Angel: "Well, I might not be locked up. You see, there are levels. If I'm on level 1 or 2, I won't get locked up."

We talked about the different levels and what it was like at the hospital. I asked her to list all of the things she did not like about the facility. She listed the food, being locked up, and that they take all of your belongings when you arrive.

> Angel: "When you go there, they take everything that is yours and they lock it up. But this time when they go to take my necklaces, I'm going to tell them to get away from me, or I'll hurt them."
> Child Life Student: "What is special about your necklaces?"
> Angel: "My boyfriend gave them to me and I don't take them off for nobody!"

I asked her if she could think of any good things about the county hospital. She immediately listed five names.

> Child Life Student: "Who are these people?"
> Angel: "The counselors."

We talked about the counselors and the sessions that she would have to attend. She mentioned a particular counselor's name several times. I suggested that perhaps this person might keep a special eye on her necklaces for her. While we were talking, she said a good thing about being hospitalized was that she could see her friends. With this remark, she smiled. She got out of bed and walked to the window. We stood there for a minute or two, talking about nothing in particular.

While standing there, we were informed that the ambulance had arrived for her. She was given the option of sedation, which she declined. Together we packed her things. I asked her if there were anything I could do that would make her transition easier. She said, "Give me something to remember you by." I suggested perhaps a note, some stickers, or a note pad. She suggested a stuffed animal. While the psychiatrist stayed with her, I left to find a stuffed animal. I returned with a small teddy bear. I explained that I had many bears myself and that I thought she might also like to have one. She took the bear and gave me a hug.

We walked out together to the hallway. The gurney arrived. She willingly got on and was strapped down. I rode the elevator with Angel to the ambulance. She was very calm and quiet. When we arrived at the ambulance, I gave her one last hug and told her that I would be thinking about her in the coming days. I could hardly believe that all this happened in less than a week and a half.

Discussion

Although Angel had many severe social and psychiatric problems, a Child Life Specialist could have ameliorated her hospital stay if more time had been available with the patient and communication with the staff had been improved. Angel was an excellent candidate for preparation for procedures. Ideally, Angel should have been prepared several hours before the procedure as well as having a nonmedical staff person present during procedures. Angel should have been given more explanations about her medical condition and its implications, and she should have been provided with the opportunity to ask questions. Even though adolescents are generally seen as "too old" for medical play, Angel, in many ways immature, might have benefited from medical play or some nonthreatening exploration of medical paraphernalia.

During her stay, Angel "selected" me to confide in about her fears and concerns. Our relationship might have allowed me to be her advocate, helping her make decisions about her care, and helping her control her anger and defensive outbursts. Such a relationship might have offset her unfortunate encounter with the young and overly challenging physician, who very much would benefit from attending Child Life rounds. Child Life also might have explored other issues of adolescence such as self-esteem, sexuality, body image, and education.

Lastly, Angel could have benefited from more one-on-one interactions with skilled adults, who could have helped her to involve herself with ward activities including socializing games with other adolescents, group painting, and board games with peers and adults. Child Life might have helped Angel develop some interpersonal skills and confidence with peers.

With more time, Child Life might have been able to show Angel and the staff the many commonalities Angel shared with other hospitalized adolescents. She might have become less a psychiatric patient and more an adolescent with whom we could work to provide quality care.

Part Four

Child Life in the Clinics

11

Child Life
in the Outpatient Department

JANETTE TACATA and BECKY HIGBY

Stanley, Age 14

Stanley, a 14-year-old African-American, came to the oncology outpatient clinic for a lumbar puncture and medication for his cancer via his mediport Broviac. The staff had labeled Stanley as "noncompliant," perhaps because of his possible gang affiliation and perhaps because the staff had little experience with adolescents.

Stanley tended to be silent and "rebellious." The staff noted that he often made the performing of procedures difficult. In short, he was an ill, unhappy adolescent. His family situation was complicated as his father was dying of cancer.

Stanley, Karen, and Carmen were reported by Janette Tacata. Becky Higby reported on her work with Roberta.

When I first introduced myself, Stanley remained silent, listening to the radio. He would not look at me or answer any questions. The nurse came to access his portacatheter. He made no attempt to comply with any requests. The nurse finally said in a stern voice, "Well, the sooner you do this the sooner it will be over. You're just making it hard on yourself, Stanley."

I asked Stanley if anything helped him through the "port access" procedure. He froze and looked at the ground. I sensed that he was afraid. When I commented that sometimes the procedure could be difficult for the patient, he let out a deep breath and worry shadowed his face. He continued to be silent and sullen. My Child Life work was limited because of the nurse's impatience with both of us. However, I found a subject that interested Stanley—basketball. Fortunately I have brothers who talk incessantly about basketball and I had experience at Camp A.O.K. (a teen camp for cancer patients). On finding this common ground, the change in Stanley's demeanor was almost magical. He told me about his team and even spoke of his favorite music. With the nurse ready for the procedure, Stanley paused, but then he removed his jacket. He said he wanted to watch. All went quickly and easily. Afterward I asked him how he felt. He shrugged his shoulders and said, "Okay." I commented that he was courageous. We continued to talk about sports, music, and dancing.

A nurse came in and explained his next procedure, a lumbar puncture (LP). Her explanation helped Stanley, and I noted how he quickly got into position for the procedure. While the doctor and nurse proceeded with the LP, I asked Stanley if he wanted me to describe what was happening or to talk about something else. He chose to talk about basketball, not wanting to know the details of what was happening. The doctor and nurse joined our conversation while they worked. Everyone seemed more relaxed, and because Stanley was cooperative no sedation was necessary. Of course, there were moments when Stanley was fearful, and I encouraged him to relax and breathe. It seemed to help that I praised him for curling up and holding still and that I followed his lead about the topic of conversation.

After the LP was completed, I acknowledged Stanley's bravery. He was able to lie still for the necessary 20 minutes as the chemotherapy took effect. I had brought Stanley's radio into the room and while we listened to music Stanley told me about his school and his clothes preferences. At one point, he stopped and said, "Listen to this song, it's my favorite." The words, "someone tell me why on earth is this the way it's supposed to be . . . I'm asking you Lord, down on bended knee," brought tears to his eyes. I was moved and unsure what to do. I said that the song was sad. Stanley made an effort to stop his tears and said, "I hate coming here." I acknowledged that it is difficult to come to the hospital. He began crying more. Sobbing he said, "I hate being sick." I listened and told him it was okay to cry. He sobbed quietly for about 10 minutes. I rubbed his arm. I thought of classes with Dr. Oremland when she said that feelings need to be felt and I did not want to interfere with his expression of them.

After a while Stanley stopped crying, and we sat quietly listening to music. I began to realize that inside this tough young man was a vulnerable child who needed support even though his actions drove us away. When I left, Stanley told me he would wear his basketball pullover next time to show me his "taste" in clothes. Later, the nurse stopped me in the hall to thank me and said, "He was a new Stanley." His mother also thanked me. I love Child Life, I thought.

I saw Stanley every week. Mostly we played card games and talked. He told me how cancer changed his life and that he missed his "gang" friends very much and felt isolated and abandoned by them.

After I completed my internship I lost contact with Stanley, although I heard that his sullenness and rebelliousness had returned. There was discussion that treatment might be stopped because of Stanley's noncompliance and missed appointments. I felt bad thinking of the limitations that being a student imposes on this work.

Karen, Age 7

Seven-year-old Karen, a Latina, had aplastic anemia. She was usually accompanied by her mother to her outpatient appointments for routine procedures and blood testing. Her mother spoke little English. Karen was generally quiet. Mostly she engaged in distraction activities such as watching videos or playing video games.

Yet, Karen also could be surprisingly verbal and able to reveal anxiety. Karen liked the nurse to tell her "when" the needle was to be injected into her arm. She was also acutely aware when a "stick" was not successful, and she often mildly scolded the nurse saying, "Try to get it right this time." Sometimes she offered a suggestion of a "good vein to use." Last week, when another girl, Ann, had an IV stick, Karen watched the entire scene unobtrusively.

I accompanied Karen on one of her IV sticks. She allowed me to hold her hand. After the procedure was completed, her nurse showered her with praise, "Good job, Karen! You did such a good job." I asked Karen how she felt. She said, "Fine. It didn't hurt." I wondered if it were true or whether she was telling me what she thought I wanted to hear. I commented that some children said that the IV starts hurt. At this point, Karen mentioned Ann. Ann was older and had cried. Karen seemed to find it incredible that an older child could engage in such "childish" behavior. I wondered if Karen might be masking her fears and decided to see if in medical play Karen could express her feelings.

Karen welcomed the prospect of medical play. She repeatedly rehearsed the blood draw, the blood testing, and the "wait" before going home. Her play was an exact reflection of her experience in the outpatient clinic. Each time, the doll, which she named Christy, was placed by "the nurse" (Karen) on her "mom's" lap (me) with her arm on the "mom's" hand or around the "mom's" neck. She said, "Christy needs" to know when the needle will enter the skin. Christy was always given the option of looking or not looking at the "stick." The doll was told to hold her breath when the needle was inside the vein and to release her breath when the needle was pulled out. This was the way Karen liked to cope with her IV procedures. I later learned that last week Karen's hands had been restrained and she was told not to look and to breathe out when the needle was inserted in the skin. For her next procedure I was able to relay Karen's preferred way of coping to her nurse.

I asked if the doll should cry and repeatedly was told that she should not cry. In time, however, Karen allowed "her baby" to cry. She then took the doll into her arms, comforted her, and talked reassuringly.

Carmen, Age 7

Carmen, a 7-year-old Latina also with aplastic anemia, had weekly appointments in the oncology outpatient clinic. For 5 weeks I provided her with play activities such as play dough, shirt painting, doll house play, and games one on one and in groups. On several occasions I supported her through procedures, generally IV sticks. Carmen developed uncontrollable bleeding and was placed in the ICU. I went to visit her, and she expressed interest in playing a board game. While we played, her nurse mentioned that Carmen had had a difficult time with injections the day before and that she was "glad to see Carmen having some fun after such a traumatic experience yesterday." I was told that Carmen recently had had multiple injections that required her to be held down while she cried and screamed.

Carmen spoke both English and Spanish, but I sensed that she preferred Spanish. Her mother spoke only Spanish. Generally quiet, Carmen communicated in many nonverbal ways including facial expression, eye contact, hesitation, stance, and smiles. I found that I had to initiate conversation with Carmen and that she would respond reluctantly with only brief answers.

Nevertheless, Carmen was receptive to play. After the board game, I asked Carmen if she wanted to play with some "special dolls." I presented two choices: playing doctor or having a tea party. I hoped to provide Carmen with medical play so that she could reenact her unhappy experience of yesterday. She chose to play doctor.

At first she was hesitant, but eventually she began taking each medical item carefully out of a bag I had brought. She neatly lined up the alcohol pads, tourniquet, adhesive bandages, arm board, stethoscope, and blood pressure cuff, looking, touching, and shaking each item and asking about the functions of some of the items. Quickly she became the "doctor." She gave the doll several injections using tourniquet, alcohol pad, adhesive bandages, and two IV sticks complete with tape and arm board. She also took a follow-up blood pressure on the doll.

Later that day, we played more board games and did art activities. Carmen became increasingly more verbal and relaxed in our play sessions. She enjoyed the challenges of the board games. I tried to speak Spanish. She enjoyed "teaching" me words and was delighted that I tried to use Spanish in our conversations. I think that my attempt at Spanish helped put Carmen's mother at ease, because she joined us in some games and taught Carmen and me how to play Solitaire.

At Carmen's request, I brought the dolls back. Carmen was now more at ease with the materials, administering many, many injections. Though she did not express personal feelings, she allowed her "baby" to cry. She was receptive to my suggestion that she hold the "baby's" hand. She asked her mother to hold the doll's hand while she counted, "uno, dos, tres" before giving the injection. In our later interactions, Carmen frequently initiated the play with the dolls and clearly and verbally expressed her preferences. Her affect range widened strikingly.

Roberta, Age 4

Four-year-old Roberta was enrolled in the Mills College Children's School, Oakland, California, where I was a student teacher. She was anxious because she was to have a "sweat test" in a hospital laboratory to rule out cystic fibrosis.

Her fear of hospitals might be related to a 1-month hospitalization of her mother a year ago. Because I had a relationship with Roberta and had completed an internship in Child Life, I was asked to help prepare Roberta for her test and accompany her during the procedure.

Roberta was of average size, had light skin, a round face, and big brown eyes. The day of the test she was nicely dressed and her long straight brown hair was perfectly styled with a matching bow. She seemed to take great pride in her appearance. Roberta was a mature 4-year-old. Her language skills were advanced, and she was inquisitive and perceptive. She enjoyed being a leader, often telling other children what to do and how to do it. Roberta was talkative and social with peers and adults.

The "sweat test" is a relatively short procedure administered by a lab technician. The child's upper arms are wrapped with a band resembling a blood pressure cuff. The arm band emits heat and pressure, thus making the child sweat. The sweat is then tested for cystic fibrosis.

Roberta's mother prepared Roberta with information about the test. While I observed, she used doll bunny rabbits to explain what would happen when at the hospital. Roberta's mother told Roberta that:

The mother bunny rabbit and the daughter bunny rabbit are going to the hospital. When they get to the hospital they see some big doors and walk in. The daughter bunny rabbit starts to feel a little afraid and the mother bunny rabbit says, "The test will go quickly. We will go into a room where a nice man or lady will wrap your arm with some gauze to make it sweat. It may feel a little warm, but it won't really hurt. The test will help the rabbit family understand why the daughter bunny rabbit has been coughing and what the family can do to make her better.

During the play, Roberta seemed somewhat interested but more concerned with eating her muffin. Yet, she did identify with the feelings of fear attributed to the daughter bunny and asked questions about how long the test would take and would the mother bunny stay with her.

After the play with the mother, Roberta and I talked. I explained that I would be at the hospital tomorrow while she had her test. She smiled and said she would like that.

Later, Roberta and I took a walk around the Children's School. She brought the bunnies on the walk and stopped on the grass to play with them. During this play, Roberta wrapped a piece of grass around the arm of the daughter bunny, explaining that she needed a test to find out why she coughed so much. At this point, she interrupted the play. I assumed that there had been enough hospital talk and followed her lead. We did not discuss the hospital further except that I later repeated to her that I would meet her the next day at the hospital.

The following day, I met Roberta and her mother in the hospital lobby. A 7-year-old girl sat next to us, and Roberta asked her why she was here. The girl's mother answered that she was there to have a "sweat test." Roberta looked at me and asked if that was the same test she was going to have. I said, "Yes." The girls exchanged a look of understanding, and I think it lessened their fears to know that other children have the same test.

On the way to the laboratory, Roberta asked many questions: where we were going, why I was there, where do I work, what would happen during the test, and if it would hurt. She seemed afraid, holding her mother's hand tightly. When we got to the laboratory's waiting room, Roberta saw a playground slide. She asked why the slide was there and if she could use it. As we waited to be called, Roberta played on the slide and seemed to be in high spirits. Yet when her name was called, the smile vanished. She immediately grabbed her mother's hand, and we followed the technician into the room.

As we walked into the small room, I explained to Roberta that the laboratory technician would tell her what he was going to do. Although he did briefly explain the procedure, he was in a hurry to start. He barely smiled at Roberta and explained that she needed to sit in the chair closest to the table. She chose to sit on her mother's lap while I sat next to them. He immediately began rubbing her arms with a liquid solution. She asked why he was doing that. He explained that he needed to clean the skin. She then asked what it was and why the cleaner was cold. We talked about why the technician was doing what he was doing and how it felt.

On the table was a mechanical device that resembled a telephone. Roberta immediately asked what the machine was and if he were going to use it on her. At this point, the technician took Roberta's arm and part of the machine that had two circular discs connected to wires. He quickly placed one disc on her arm and then wrapped it with another part of the machine that resembled a blood pressure cuff. He repeated the same process with the other arm. Roberta became upset and began to cry, exclaiming that no one told her there was going to be a "stupid" machine.

I explained that this machine was going make her skin warm so she would sweat. I encouraged her to talk about how it felt and validated her feelings regarding not knowing what was going to happen. I said, "It's scary when you don't know what is going to happen and that you didn't know about this machine. I bet the man could tell us exactly what this machine does.'

The technician took my cue and told Roberta that the arm cuff might feel a bit tight and warm and that it would remain on her arm for 6 minutes. Given her age and inability to grasp the concept of time in minutes, Roberta asked, "How long is 6 minutes?" I reassured her, giving her a time frame to which she could relate. "About as long as it takes to read your favorite book," I said.

Roberta cried during the 6 minutes. Over and over she said, "I hate the stupid machine." She complained that it was too hot and squeezed her arm. I addressed these issues with her and attempted to validate her feelings in a supportive and informative manner.

I let Roberta know that she was doing a good job, and I kept emphasizing that "pretty soon" the test would be over and the man would take the cuffs off her arms. I asked, "I'm wondering if there is something we could do to make the time go by faster?" She suggested that we read the story she brought, which we read twice. During this time she asked questions like, "How much longer? Why is it squeezing my arm so tightly? Why is it so hot?" Again I attempted to address her questions in a supportive manner providing accurate and age-appropriate information.

As soon as the test was over, the technician applied a strip of gauze to the reddened areas on her arms. He then added more gauze and tape to hold the strips in place. He explained that we could leave the testing room and return in 20 minutes to remove the bandages. Roberta commented on the fact that her arms were red but that she felt much better now that the machine was off. She included, "It wasn't so bad. I just didn't like the machine part."

Roberta repeatedly talked about the fact that no one had told her about the machine and how much she hated it. I explained that her mother and I did not know about the machine either.

While we waited, we talked about what was going to happen next. She repeatedly asked, "Are you sure they are just going to remove the bandages and that is all?" as if she felt unsure given our lack of knowledge regarding the machine part of the test. I continued to reassure her, and we talked about exactly what would happen. She worried about the hurt when the tape came off. I told her, "The tape is a special kind of tape that hurts a little but less than when you take a Band-Aid off." We talked about what she could do to make the bandage removal better for her, and she came up with the idea of taking the bandage off very slowly. I told her we could make this suggestion to the technician.

We went to the cafeteria and Roberta saw the same girl from the lobby, who also had bandaged arms. Roberta immediately told the girl, "I didn't like the machine. You have a bandage just like mine." The two girls compared bandages, and Roberta said, "I'm going to get mine off soon and so will you." The girl's mother told us that her daughter did not like the machine either. The girls looked at each other in knowing silence.

When we returned to the laboratory I said, "Roberta, did you remember what you wanted to tell the man?" Roberta said to the technician, "I want you to take the bandage off very slowly." He replied, "Well, it will hurt less if I go fast." I said, "Why don't we let Roberta decide. Which would you rather have Roberta, fast or slow?" She replied, "slow." He began to take the bandages off slowly, speeding up at the end. Roberta appeared somewhat empowered by the control she gained in deciding the speed at which the bandages would be removed.

She watched carefully as he removed the gauze strip and placed it in a sterile bottle. Her mother and I explained that they were taking the strip of gauze to the laboratory to look at her sweat. Roberta commented once again, "This wasn't so bad. I just didn't like the machine part." As we walked out the door and down the hallway Roberta was in high spirits. She talked about the treat her mom promised her.

Discussion of Roberta

Accompanying Roberta during her diagnostic procedure provided an unusual opportunity to understand the laboratory experience that children encounter when they come to the hospital for a testing procedure. As in Roberta's case, children often are faced with the hospital setting for the first time, an anxiety-laden experience.

The laboratory technicians in general seemed rushed and not very thoughtful with the children or adults, rarely taking time for conversation or explanation. This attitude clearly has a negative influence on the experience of a child coming into the hospital environment for the first time.

The interaction between Roberta and the other young girl was interesting. They were comforted by the knowledge that they shared the same experience. In addition, Roberta was somewhat empowered by the fact that she went through the test first, reassuring the girl that the bandages would be coming off soon. Lastly, this experience reaffirmed the importance of relaying accurate information in the preparation of any medical experience a child may face, regardless of how minor it may be. As was seen with Roberta, when a child does not experience exactly what he or she is expecting, anxiety can increase. Roberta's experience reminds us that even under the best of circumstances and with a thoughtful, careful mother and expert preparation these experiences are at the least trying and at the most traumatic to young children.

12

Child Life
in an Infusion Unit

JO LEE

Lilly, Age 6

Lilly, a 6-year-old African-American with sickle cell disease, had suffered a stroke 2 years earlier leaving her with severe left-sided sensorineural hearing loss and global deficits in cognitive development. She received special education services at school and was on a strict medical protocol with blood transfusions every 3 weeks in the Infusion Unit. Her grandmother brought her for the treatments and was her primary caregiver.

I first met Lilly at a Sickle Cell Family Information Evening when she was 5 years old—everyone participated except Lilly. At that time she was 1 year poststroke and incapable of focusing on an activity. A year later, she was like a humming bird, flitting from one thing to the next. She laughed all the while and seemed to be having a wonderful time. It was hard to imagine that this child was the same little girl. The staff of the Infusion Unit wanted the grandmother to start Lilly on chelation therapy at home. Both Lilly and the grandmother were hesitant to begin this treatment, and I was asked by the unit's manager to work with the family to ease their fears about performing the treatment at home. It was also planned that I would see Lilly when she came to the Infusion Unit for her blood transfusions.

Chelation therapy helps patients who are chronically transfused dissipate the iron that accumulates in the tissues. The therapy is a simple procedure that continues so long as the transfusions are needed. It can often be an overwhelming prospect for the child and the parents.

Chelation therapy entails placing a needle 0.5 centimeters long under the skin. For most children the fleshy part of their abdomen is an ideal location. The medication is then infused into the body using a 5-inch, battery-powered pump. Many children are infused at night.

I discovered that even though the procedure had been carefully explained to the grandmother, the explanation had taken place without using actual materials. When the Infusion Unit nurse had talked about "the pump," the grandmother had imagined an enormous contraption. The imagery was frightening. It was not surprising that she was resistant to being responsible. I had access to all the equipment so I was able to show the grandmother how the pump worked. Her fear lessened when I explained that a team of professionals would make home visits to help her with each step of the treatment until she felt comfortable administering the medication alone.

Lilly's grandmother usually brought her to the Infusion Unit for her transfusion. The same nurse began all the treatments, and Lilly and she developed a rapport. From experience both Lilly and the nurse knew which of Lilly's veins

were most suitable for her IV. Nevertheless, Lilly always reminded the nurse where she wanted the IV. Children often
know which veins work best for their IV. She also liked to be
talked to during the process of having the medicine injected.

Generally when Lilly arrived at the Infusion Unit she had
breakfast and frequently asked to do medical play. Her play
was active, mostly consisting of giving IV's and shots to a doll.

Lilly usually came for her transfusion on Mondays. One
time she had to come on a Friday and the grandmother,
who had an appointment, had to leave Lilly alone. That
morning her usual nurse was unavailable. Two nurses, Maggie and Sue, one of whom Lilly knew and liked, began her
transfusion.

Lilly was calm as the nurses began the IV. Maggie and Sue
inserted the needle but did not find the vein. Lilly remained
calm. The second attempt also failed. Lilly became anxious.
Maggie asked me to join them. I sat next to Lilly to let her
know how brave she was being and how hard it was when
the IV did not work the first time. I let her know she could
hold onto my hand and squeeze it if she wanted to. She did
and began to cry as the nurses inserted the butterfly needle
for the third time. When the third attempt failed the needle
was withdrawn, and the nurses began to discuss the possibili-
ties of using the "big needle." This was prepared, and the
nurses took hold of Lilly's arm. They thought that the veins
on her forearm looked promising, even though Lilly liked
them to use the veins on the top of her hands. The nurses
looked at me. One said, "We're just going to do it."

Lilly became nearly hysterical, and I told the nurses that
we should stop briefly. I wanted to talk to Lilly about the
needles and see if she wanted some medical play. Unfortunately Sue and I did not know each other, and neither of
the nurses was pleased with my suggestion. Maggie looked
at me and said, "You have 15 minutes."

Lilly fell into my body and cried. We just hugged for a
while, and I let her know how hard it must be when things

do not work the way you want them to. I let her know that I wanted to talk about the different needles and maybe do some medical play. Lilly said over and over, "I want the butterfly. I want the butterfly." I responded, "I know you want the butterfly needle, Lilly, but sometimes, because the veins get tired, the butterflies do not work as well. I know the blue needle (I did not want to say the big needle) looks different and it may even look a little longer, but really it's just as small as the butterfly. You know it looks different too, because there is a little piece of white plastic that goes over the needle." I wondered if she had seen this difference. She nodded, "Yes." I continued, "When the nurse sets up your IV with the blue needle the white cover stays on. Once everything is in place, she will take out the needle so that only the white plastic stays in the vein." Lilly was still crying, but less so than before. She clung tightly to me.

There was a pause, and then she suddenly blurted out very quickly, "I got poked in my private parts, a shot in my private parts." For a moment terrible thoughts passed through my mind. I remained calm. "Where did this happen, Lilly? Was it at home or in the hospital?" I asked. I realized that this was a directed question, but I thought it was important to get the details. "In the hospital," she wept. "That sounds as if it were very upsetting for you, Lilly," I replied. "In my private parts," she wept. We sat and cuddled. I wondered if the mention of the big needle had evoked a previous memory of a physically painful experience.

Lilly suddenly wanted medical play. We got out the dolls and the real needles. I only had a butterfly needle, so I showed her with the butterfly how the plastic was the part that stayed in the vein and how the needle came out. I told her that Seb, the little boy in the bed opposite, had a blue needle. I asked her if she wanted to see it. She said, "Yes." Seb was pleased to show her his IV, and he told her that she should get one, too. He wanted to join Lilly and do some medical play. I noted a lessening of anxiety. I sat back and watched. The children began to laugh and exchange words and ideas. They set up IV's, put on Band-Aids, and gave lots of shots. At one point Lilly pulled away from the medical play and sat on Seb's bed to play Nintendo.

Of course this intervention took longer than 15 minutes. Maggie approached me. "We are going to use the 'big needle,' " she said. I let them know that Lilly was ready for them to use the *other* needle and that I had called it the "blue needle." Lilly came over and sat on her bed putting out her arm. Sue told her she was going to use the "blue needle." Lilly did not move. She watched intensely and asked me for my hand. She squeezed my hand as the needle went into the vein. The first try was successful. Lilly turned to me and said, "You did not lie." She looked at Maggie and Sue and said, "I do not ever want a butterfly needle again, I want a blue one like Seb has." Maggie and Sue said that they would be sure to remember that for the next time. I turned to Lilly, gave her a hug, and told her how brave she had been.

When I returned to the office, the nurses were buzzing with excitement over what had taken place. I thought now would be a good opportunity to talk to the staff about choice of words when dealing with children. We talked about the perceptions of a child relative to the "butterfly" versus the "big" needle. I suggested that perhaps the imagery that these two words conjured up for a child were extreme. Even an adult would have difficulty understanding the benefits of the "big" needle when compared to a "butterfly." I explained to the staff why I had chosen to use the word *blue* to describe the needle. The needle has a blue plastic covering at the end away from the needle. Focusing on the color "blue" may have helped Lilly not to focus on the needle itself. A nurse or doctor could perhaps use the color blue to help the child visualize the beautiful blue colors that they see in their lives. The team was very responsive and agreed.

I also needed to mention Lilly's idea about "the shot in my private parts." The chart showed that she had recently undergone her first catherization and that must have been frightening to her. It upset the staff to realize Lilly's misperception of the events.

Seb, Age 6

Seb was a 6-year-old Laotian boy diagnosed with Hemoglobin E Beta Thalassemia, a chronic anemia typically found by age 1 month in individuals of Southeast Asian and Mediterranean descent. He was born prematurely at 28 weeks and had been transfused regularly since he was 18 months.

Staff members told me that various adults accompanied Seb to the Infusion Unit. Sometimes he was simply dropped off. On the morning I met Seb, he was accompanied by his grandmother, who was not feeling well and went to lie down. Seb spoke fluent English.

The nursing staff requested that I work with Seb as the boy often required four or five people to hold him while he was set up with his IV. Seb showed no real sign of wanting to talk to me. Obviously he was an angry little boy ready to fight. I offered him play dough. He did not speak to me. I began talking, saying that play dough was "pretty good stuff" for molding, slapping on the table, and even banging against the wall. Seb waited until I had left before he began slapping and pummeling the play dough. He threw it at the wall, put it on the floor, and stamped on it.

On our next meeting, I reminded Seb that he seemed to enjoy playing with the play dough last time and wondered if he would like to play with some again. Seb said, "No!" without looking away from his Nintendo. I continued, "I also remember how upset you were when the nurse set you up with your IV. I wondered if it made you feel angry?" "Yes," he said. He added, "It makes me mad." I continued, "I wonder if you would like to put an IV on a doll?" I had barely finished talking when he said, "Yes."

I took out a doll and a box of medical equipment that I had brought. Seb opened the box and took out the tape. He tore off a piece and put it over the doll's mouth. "I wonder why your baby needs tape over his mouth?" I asked. "Because he screams," he replied. Seb took the Betadine sticks that are placed on the skin to promote anesthesia and poked them into the doll's eyes. Next he attached the IV board to the doll's arm. He rubbed on more Betadine. "I wonder if the baby is scared?" I asked. "Yes," he replied, "but he's mad too." "What would make him less scared?" I inquired. "I do not know," he said. He lifted up the doll's shirt and began to rub the Betadine on the baby's tummy. "Is that where he gets his desferral?" "Yes," he said. He lifted up his shirt and showed me his tummy. "You have a desferral too?" I asked. He nodded.

I asked him if he would like me to stay with him when the nurses set him up for the IV. He said, "Yes." I told him that I was going to let the nurse know that I would stay with him.

I went to the office to tell the nurse about Seb's extreme anger. Then I returned to Seb. As the nurse prepared the IV, Seb gave her his arm. She put on the tourniquet. Seb was obviously unhappy with his situation, but he cooperated.

When the nurse indicated she was ready to insert the needle Seb shouted. I gave him my hand. He squeezed it very tightly, but he otherwise was still. The needle entered the vein the first time. The nurse commented on how brave Seb had been and how it was all right to feel angry and shout when he got his IV.

"How do you feel now, Seb?" she asked. "Mad," he said. I reiterated how brave he had been and remarked on how he had been able to "keep still" all by himself. It was gratifying to see how he was able to express himself and then positively participate in his treatment.

In our next session, Seb continued his angry behavior, often hitting the play dough and doing lots of medical play, especially with real needles. At the end of the session for the first time he asked for crayons. He made a card for me. No longer did he require the four or five people to hold him down. He would keep very still during procedures, and he was indeed proud of himself.

Danielle, Age 10

Danielle, a 10-year-old African-American, was diagnosed with sickle cell disease when she was 6 months old. She suffered a severe stroke at age 3 that left her with slurred speech, right-sided weakness, and cognitive functioning in the low range.

Danielle lived with her aunt. Her mother had a history of drug use. Her living conditions had been reported as "chaotic." Danielle began regular transfusions every 4 weeks at age 6. The aunt worked 7 days a week, and she and Danielle traveled a long distance by bus, so there were great difficulties in Danielle's coming for treatment.

On a day that Danielle was admitted for a "total exchange," a potentially dangerous procedure that required admission to the ICU, the aunt explained that they were already tired from the long bus ride. I knew Danielle from numerous previous admissions, and I let her know that I would come with her to the ICU. We waited a long time for a bed to become available, and I was getting worried knowing that I would have to leave relatively soon.

At last we heard that there was a bed. I did not know what to expect in that I had never accompanied a child to the ICU, a sterile environment with many very sick children.

As soon as we entered the ICU, Danielle's aunt said that she needed to make a phone call. Her aunt was clearly overwhelmed by the very sick children that surrounded us. She could not stop herself from commenting on how they looked and how she could not stand it. I tried to acknowledge her feelings about this overwhelming environment. I attempted to change the subject, as I did not think it was helping Danielle to focus on the other children. The aunt left.

Danielle told me that she had been there before. "This is the bed I was in when I had my stroke," she said anxiously. I tried to reassure her that she would be all right and empathized with how difficult it must be to come back to this unit. I assured her that today she was not going to be here long and that she and her aunt would be going home today. The nurses had told me that the exchange would take just about the same length of time as a normal transfusion. I shared this information with Danielle.

The nurse approached Danielle's bed. She told her that she needed to get undressed and put on a gown. Tears began to trickle down Danielle's face. I was confused too. She had been admitted as an outpatient. The children in the Infusion Unit do not undress. I asked the nurse if it were really necessary for Danielle to change her clothes? She said that it was, adding "just in case there is a blood spill." Danielle did not want to change. I acknowledged how difficult it was to have plans changed. I reassured her that putting on the gown did not mean she would be staying at the hospital. I added that if it made her feel better, she could keep her clothes close to her bed. She continued to cry, hold on to me, and undressed very slowly.

The nurse told her that she was going to put some numbing cream on her arms. I explained that the numbing cream would help take away the pain when the IV's were placed. The nurse spread the cream on four separate areas, two on the wrists and two on the creases of the forearms. Danielle began to cry again. "They're going to put four needles in me," she wept. "Danielle," I said calmly, "you remember Maury in the Infusion Unit this morning?" She nodded. "Remember how he had two needles in his arms? That's what you will have, just two needles." I explained that the nurse put the numbing cream on four places to see where the needle could best be inserted. I reminded her that sometimes the nurses cannot find a vein right away, so they have to look in another area. She stopped crying and lay on the bed. She asked for a blanket, an extra one so she could lie on top of the bed instead of climbing into it. I wrapped her, and she molded her body next to mine. We watched television, and she told me about the different rock groups she knew.

I realized that I would not be able to stay with Danielle during her treatment as the numbing medicine needed an hour to take effect. I wondered why this part of the procedure had not been done downstairs in the familiar surrounding of the Infusion Unit.

Danielle was comfortable when I left. I found her aunt in the Infusion Unit. I told her that I was leaving and that Danielle was alone in the ICU.

Later I found out that Danielle did not come back from the ICU until late in the afternoon. She became so upset during the procedure that she had to be heavily sedated. When she returned to the Infusion Unit she was still incapable of standing. Her aunt had only briefly visited her during the procedure and then had returned to the Infusion Unit.

I saw Danielle approximately 2 months later when she returned to the Infusion Unit with her aunt. She was wrapped in bed covers and looked despondent. I knew Danielle would be at the unit that day, and I remembered to bring her a letter that she had written and decorated for her teacher the last time she had been here. I showed her the letter and told her I had saved it for her. She immediately sat up and wanted to write more letters.

She was apprehensive when it was time to start the IV. She said she wanted a mediport, which the sickle cell team had been encouraging her to have since the episode in the ICU. Danielle began to cry because the nurses wanted to use the "big" needle. I went to sit with her and tried to clarify that the needles looked different but in fact were the same length. Danielle nodded. I put my arm around her and told her she could hold me tightly if she wanted. She did. She began to panic as the needle pierced the skin. I suggested that she blow away the hurt. She did. The needle went in the first time. The nurses taped the area securely so that she did not have to have a board.

Yasmina, Age 13

Yasmina, a 13-year-old African-American, was about 100 to 150 pounds overweight. She had secondary health problems including kidney failure due to her obesity. She came to the Infusion Unit for a series of tests and treatments, each of which took about 2 hours. She was given medication intravenously, hooked up to a monitor, and blood was taken every 30 minutes.

Yasmina was generally accompanied by her mother and her aunt. The family was very religious. I watched the mother and aunt retreat for long periods to a small annex to pray.

Yasmina was a reserved, sedentary child who rarely spoke. Her voice was high pitched, babylike. Previously, she had only wanted to play Nintendo, but one day she asked to paint. As I sat with her, she proceeded to paint many different-colored dots on yellow paper. She liked the yellow paper and kept asking for more. I asked if she painted at school or at home. She responded "No." At our next meeting, Yasmina wanted to paint again and continued making dots. She stayed close to me all morning.

Later in the week when Yasmina returned for treatment, she announced that she wanted to paint but that she did not want to paint any more dots. Andrew, an 8-year-old boy, wanted to join in, and she agreed. So Andrew sat down and started to paint too. The differences between the two children were remarkable. Andrew loved to experiment. He painted large images. He loved to pour and mix. Yasmina worked very neatly, very slowly, and very deliberately. She watched Andrew's frenzied movements—perhaps in wonder, perhaps in horror. Yasmina seemed incapacitated by Andrew's style. Andrew quickly left, and Yasmina decided to make a pattern. Her movements were small and hesitant. Largely she cut paper into strips and glued them on the page in an orderly fashion.

The next week Yasmina again wanted to paint. She added, "I'm going to do something else today." She painted two houses. "This is the mommy house, and this is the baby house," she said. She then cut out paper flowers, painted them, and stuck them on to the page next to the houses. Her process was more advanced than before but not at the level of a 13-year-old. Her doctor interrupted the play with several medical questions. Yasmina's mother had just arrived and was trying to encourage Yasmina to describe the tingling sensations she had been having in her back.

When the doctor left, I tried to encourage Yasmina to speak for herself. "You know it's all right to tell the doctor what you have been experiencing. You are the one who knows best, because it's your body," I said. When the doctor returned, Yasmina explained hesitantly the sensations she had been having. The doctor asked about school. She said she had not attended school for 10 days. When asked why, she told the doctor that she had been feeling weak.

I decided to try to find out more about Yasmina. To help her I thought it would be beneficial to know what was happening at school, with friends, and at home. I wondered why whenever I came to see Yasmina she always asked her mother and aunt to leave.

When we next met, Yasmina was busy with Nintendo. I suggested we talk. When I asked her about school, her voice changed and lost its baby quality. She told me she liked spelling and had won awards for being the best in academics. I was surprised to hear these comments from a reticent youngster who gave few clues as to her capabilities. She told me that her school required parents to volunteer 40 hours per year to help the school. She told me that her mother was too busy with her church to fulfill her obligations so Yasmina performed the school service for her mother in the school cafeteria. She added that she very much liked working there. I did not mention the food aspect of this activity, as she heard a lot about overeating from everyone else.

When I asked Yasmina about schoolfriends, she said she had one girl friend but they only saw each other at school. I wondered aloud about when she was planning to return to school. She replied that she had many choir practices at church to consider first.

Yasmina brought up the subject of her grandmother. "Do you see your granny a lot?" I asked. "I live with her," she said. "My mommy's boyfriend used to hit me, so my granny came to get me when I was 5 years old." "That must have been hard for you," I said. She began painting. "Can you keep a secret?" she said. "What kind of secret?" I asked. "Something one of the ladies at the church told me," she continued. "The lady told me that something very terrible had happened to me and one day I would be able to talk to my mother about it. Guess what it is?" she pushed. I asked her if it had something to do with her granny's coming to get her? She replied, "Yes." "Do you want to tell me what it is?" I asked. "No, I want you to guess. My mom told me I'm not supposed to tell anyone." I asked if it were something painful? "Yes," she said. "Do you want to tell me what it is?" I asked. "My mom's boyfriend molested me. That's what the lady at the church said." I asked her if she remembered when it happened? She said, "No." I asked her if she had spoken to her granny about it. She said, "Yes, but granny didn't know for sure. She just had a funny feeling about him. That's why she came to get me."

I asked Yasmina if she had talked to her counselor about this matter. She said, "No, it's a secret." While we were talking, Yasmina stopped painting and picked up a banana from her breakfast tray. She painted it purple.

I was unsure about going further. I discussed the conversation with a consultant who said that the incident must be reported to Child Protective Services. I wanted to talk to Yasmina's social worker, someone who Yasmina had told me she liked. I asked the social worker if Yasmina had been told about possible abuse. The social worker stated that she had inquired and the mother was adamant that nothing had happened.

The social worker and the consultant wanted me to tell Yasmina that I had to report the incident. Reluctant to do so, I explained that I wanted to give Yasmina the opportunity to tell the social worker herself so as not to breach her confidence. I explained to Yasmina that the information she had told me was important and that she needed to tell someone who would be able to help her explore what happened. I wondered if she would be willing to tell her social worker. To my amazement, she said, "Yes." I asked her if she wanted me to stay or leave while she talked with the social worker. She asked me to stay. As her conversation deepened with the social worker, she began to hesitate. I asked her if she wanted me to leave. She nodded a "yes."

Maddy, Age 3

Maddy, a 3-year-old Arab girl, suffered from Factor VIII deficiency, a rare factor deficiency causing lifelong coagulopathy characterized by delayed bleeding that may occur several days after an injury. Maddy was seen monthly in the Infusion Unit. Each month she was given what the medical team called "a push," a 15- to 20-minute period during which prophylactic medicines were given intravenously. She returned home when the treatment was completed.

The head nurse informed me that Maddy did not cope at all well with her treatments, becoming rigid and screaming uncontrollably. At least three people were required to hold her for her "push."

The day I met Maddy she arrived at the unit with her father, her 5-year-old sister, and an uncle. Maddy clung to her father. I introduced myself to the family. Not wanting to scare Maddy, I directed the invitation to play to her sister, and I suggested that Maddy come and join us once she had been weighed. Her sister was enthusiastic and spoke to Maddy in Arabic. Maddy began to whimper. She did not want to be weighed.

Once the medical preliminaries were over, I asked Maddy again if she would like to play. She shook her head, "No." When I showed her some play dough, she took it out of my hand. Her father spoke to her in Arabic and then in English. He made a figure of a baby in the play dough, which she liked. She then moved to join her sister at the table. Not long after, the father told me that he had to leave, adding that he never stayed when Maddy had her treatment. I asked if she knew he were leaving and if he had said good-bye. He said that she knew he would be leaving and that he did not want her to cry. The father explained, "If I stay, she cries. If I leave she doesn't." Remembering that the nurses had told me that Maddy cried unconsolably when her father was not there, I wondered if it were too hard for him to witness her distress.

The two sisters remained engaged with the play dough for about 15 minutes and then asked to play with something else. I introduced the idea of the dolls and medical play. I wondered if they would like to practice putting an IV on the dolls. Both were eager.

Maddy's sister told me how her baby needed to get a shot, but before she got it she needed to have tape over her mouth. I asked, "Why?" She replied, "Because she cries so much." Maddy put Band-Aid after Band-Aid on the doll's mouth but would not touch the syringes, even though her sister tried to encourage her on numerous occasions. These syringes were of the same type that the nurses used for the "push."

I asked Maddy if her baby needed to go to the hospital to get medicine. She answered, "Yes." I wondered aloud if it were frightening for her. She replied, "Yes." She picked up her baby and gave her a hug and a kiss. I reflected that she was taking good care of her baby. At this moment the father peeked into the unit. The children could not see him. He quickly disappeared when he saw that Maddy was still waiting for her treatment.

Maddy's sister wanted to be with the father. I took her to the waiting area, but he had gone. I was torn. I did not want to leave the sister there unsupervised, yet I wanted to be with Maddy.

I left the 5-year-old in the waiting area and returned to Maddy. She was sitting quietly having her "push." The nurse appeared and said she was all done. She added, "Maddy had offered her arm and remained relaxed all during the 'push.' " Maddy announced, "It didn't hurt."

When the father returned, I told him how brave Maddy had been and how she had not cried. I was tempted to discuss his leaving with him, but he went on, "I know. That's why I leave. Then she doesn't cry." I thought it was best to leave him with his idea. It appeared that leaving the room was the only way he could deal with his distress.

Maddy turned to me before she left. She flung her arms around my neck, and I received a big kiss.

Kayla, Age 14

Kayla, a 14-year-old African-American, was diagnosed with systemic lupus erythematosus (SLE—Lupus) and lupus-related nephrites at age 12. She had been receiving chemotherapy in the Infusion Unit for about 18 months. Her therapy began early in the morning each day of her treatment and continued for about 12 hours. Later in the day she was transferred to an inpatient floor where she completed her treatment and spent the night. Kayla did not like the overnight stays.

I spent one enchanting morning with Kayla. She was lying on her bed watching television as I approached. She flicked through the channels, not taking her eyes from the screen. Her face looked empty and uninterested. I introduced myself and finished my sentence with, "If you would just like to talk, that would be fine too."

Immediately she sat up and said, "I'd like to talk." She turned off the television and turned to face me. She was an innocent-looking young girl with a captivating smile. I asked her about her treatment program. She said that she would be staying overnight and that she had brought some homework with her. She brought out a French book. She was excited that she had started taking French this year. I told her I had lived in France and that I spoke French. I added that if she wanted, we could practice French together. She liked the idea and began to read in French. Her accent was beautiful, and she was at ease as she practiced her grammar and pronunciation.

When Kayla finished with the French homework, she brought out more books from her school bag. One of her books was a novel by C. S. Lewis, *The Voyage of the Dawn Treader*. She began to retell one of the passages that she had enjoyed. She sat back in her bed looking as though she could see the small boat sailing toward the sun that she was describing to me. She spoke of how the water glistened as the boat bobbed. She closed her eyes as if to see the image more clearly. Her account was beautiful. It was magical, just as Lewis had meant it to be.

She asked me about other things she had read about in Lewis' books, such as pigeon pie and Turkish Delight. In that I am English, I knew exactly how to describe these English foods to her. Kayla also had noticed that some of Lewis' English spellings were different from American spelling.

Kayla had brought other books with her, some she had had since she was 10 years old. It seemed that these books had been with her since the time of her diagnosis. She brought the books with her each time she came to the hospital, rather like transitional objects. I wondered if they reminded her of a life less complicated, evoking memories of healthier times. She had passages memorized from each of her books, and she knew where to find each passage in the book without pause for thought. When she read to me, I felt she was sharing a part of herself.

When Kayla's doctor arrived, we were discussing Lewis. The doctor did not interrupt. He too was familiar with Lewis, and he joined in our conversation. He sat down and spoke softly and respectfully. I introduced myself to him and then excused myself. I let Kayla know that I would be back. I thanked the doctor for being patient with our discussion and responding to Kayla in such a warm way.

Later that morning Kayla wanted to attend a puppet show in the inpatient playroom. We sat side by side. Kayla was enthralled by the show and laughed a lot. When the show was over, she wanted to remain in the playroom. She made her way over to the play dough. I was surprised that she wanted to play. It was often hard for teenagers to allow themselves to regress even a little. She was able to express frustrations in this play. She hit the play dough and banged it hard on the table. She smashed it and pummeled it without words. When it was time to close the playroom for the lunch period, she was sad to leave.

We returned to the unit and Kayla talked about her family. She was the middle of five children. She described her place in the family in relation to her other siblings. According to Kayla, if you were the eldest you could do what you liked. If you were the youngest, you got all the attention. "The one in the middle is just there," she said.

We talked about friends and school. She told me that she felt short and fat. The steroids she took as part of her medical protocol gave her face a bloated appearance and gave her a distended abdomen. However, she was still a lovely young woman.

Food entered the conversation. Kayla was supposed to follow a strict salt-free diet. She told me that the only time she really followed the diet was when she came to the hospital. It worried me that Kayla was unaware that by not complying with the dietary instructions, she was, in fact, putting her life at greater risk. Many interesting conversations followed.

Part Five

The School-Age Child

13

Summer and the School-Age Child in the Hospital

Lauren Manheimer

Child Life programs effectively reach many age groups. During the day the playroom is populated by toddlers and preschool children who engage in onlooker play, solitary independent activities, and associative art projects in coordination with adults. In the evenings, adolescents frequently are involved in games in a Teen Lounge. Yet casual observation raises a question: Where are the school-age children between the ages of 6 and 12? What can Child Life offer this population of children, particularly during the summer months when there is no school program?

Harry

I encouraged Harry, age 10, to come to the playroom for a birthday party and some board games. In the playroom, he seemed uncharacteristically quiet and withdrawn, and he was eager to return to his room. He explained, "I just feel uncomfortable around all those little kids. It's like I don't belong . . . and I'm not old enough for the Teen Lounge, even though I know they do cool stuff in there. . . . Last time I was here I could at least hang out with kids my own age in the school program."

It was summertime, and Harry confirmed my suspicion that school-age children were "falling through the cracks." He had raised a critical question. Ten months of the year a school program serves as a special sanctuary in the hospital for school-age children. Each day they temporarily escape the medical environment and enter a space of social interactions among age-mates in school-related activities. The acquisition of new skills and friends is exceedingly important to the school-age child. With illness and hospitalization, concerns of falling behind academically and being abruptly cut off from family and peer relationships are marked and disruptive. A program specifically designed for school-age children can act as a buffer against such psychological distress by fostering competence, belonging, control, and mastery.

Christopher

My time with Christopher, a 9-year-old sickle cell patient, further underscored the need for a school-age program during the summer months. Christopher's chronic illness necessitated frequent hospitalizations. I noticed a dramatic change in his behavior during a hospitalization in July in comparison with a previous hospitalization.

One afternoon, I visited Christopher. He informed me that like Harry he did not feel that he belonged in the playroom. I explained to him that the playroom is a play place for children of all ages and that there were many activities suitable for 9-year-olds. He plainly declared that he did not "enjoy" being a part of it. Christopher conveyed his personal meaning of "summer" and how hospitalization during this time was particularly distressing. Like many children, Christopher saw summer as an opportunity for outdoor play, swimming, fun, laughter among friends, and no homework.

For chronically ill schoolchildren, however, summer in the sense of freedom, is suddenly taken away and replaced by sickness and dreadful longing. Hospitalization during the summer months poses a particular threat to the psychosocial well-being of school-age children. A specific summer program can provide essential ways to cope with difficult feelings associated with the bitterness of summertime illness. Group play among peers may promote self-expression and a sense of belonging. Further, a specific school-age program during the summer months can foster learning, competence, and self-esteem in school-age children.

Developmental Issues in the School-Age Child

The literature tells us that the school ages represent the least vulnerable period for hospitalization of children (Eckenhoff, 1953; James, 1960). The literature asserts that during this time the child has largely mastered fears of separation and abandonment and is not yet struggling with the exaggerated need of adolescents to be independent. Nonetheless, the school-age child harbors significant developmental concerns that must be understood if we are to design an effective Child Life program for all children.

The growth of the school-age child (ages 6 to 12) is slow and steady until the preadolescent growth spurt. These middle years represent a time of consolidation of perceptions of self and other with developing competence, self-assurance, and social abilities that will allow eventual independence from the family. Jean Piaget has termed this period the stage of *concrete operations* of thought and interpersonal relations (Piaget & Inhelder, 1969, pp. 92–129). The concrete operational child has developed the ability to perceive another's point of view and comprehend the meaning of a series of actions. Therefore, "A child of this age is better able to understand a thorough preparation for surgery or procedures, including all of the steps entailed in the process" (Thompson & Stanford, 1981, p. 71). "He has also become more adept in using symbols in order to express himself verbally, to write, and to read. . . . He acquires the basic concepts of numbers, weight, time, space and speed" (Lindheim, Glaser, & Coffin, 1972, p. 57). The school-age child's increasing ability to reason logically, sequence events, and impose order is directly reflected in play. The focus shifts from the exploratory process of interacting with materials to play with preconceived goals that emphasizes some end-product. "Games and other activities founded upon rules predominate. Secret clubs are established, based on well-planned charters. Teams are formed, and group activities become more competitive than in previous years" (Thompson & Stanford, 1981, p. 71).

Physically, school-age children have gained considerable motor coordination that enables them to practice skills and develop strengths in a variety of athletic games and crafts. Accomplishments of numerous tasks award the child a critical sense of competence and control. "Around nine years old, some enjoy being responsible for what they do and will often plan and carry out complicated projects with such things as model making or scientific experiments" (Harvey & Hales-Tooke, 1972, p. 68).

At the same time, school-age children form their first mutual friendships and learn to work cooperatively in a group setting through ongoing communication and negotiation.

In fact, the school-age child's social–emotional world becomes centered around peer interactions, although the children remain highly dependent on family support. Frequently, school-age children prefer friends of the same sex. From a developmental standpoint, this is essential in promoting an understanding of self. Together, the same-sex friends may engage in dramatic play in which they act out social rules and roles with costumes and props. The fact that the influence of friends rivals the influence of parents and other adults is evidence of the immeasurable importance of the peer group at this time of development (Lindheim et al., 1972).

Hospitalization and Illness

Illness and hospitalization in school-age children often produce ongoing, regressive dependency on family and an inability to develop age-appropriate skills at the same pace as peers. Although these children may have made marked advances in their ability to reason logically, they are still likely to use fantasy to fill the gaps in their understanding. They may harbor feelings of guilt or self-blame for their illness, despite an increasing ability to comprehend the causality of disease.

> The image of parents as benevolent guardians is challenged by reality when the child sees his parents helpless to protect him from suffering. He may even imagine that he is being punished for misdeeds by being hospitalized and separated from the warmth and support of his family. The sick child reacts to these real and imagined situations with increased dependency, regression, and anxiety. (Lindheim et al., 1972, p. 58)

Feelings of loss of body integrity in addition to restrictions of mobility may severely threaten the school-age child's newly acquired sense of mastery as maintained through physical activity. "Whereas the healthy school-age child takes his body for granted, illness produces a heightened and uncomfortable concern about physiological functions and forces the child to cope prematurely with concepts of illness and death" (Lindheim et al., 1972, p. 58).

In conjunction with the aggravated fear of isolation, loss of control, incompetence, and mutilation, abrupt separation from peers and family can bring debilitating psychological distress with feelings of abandonment, insecurity, and distrust. Group play and ongoing preparation are effective means of enhancing the child's feelings of competence and control. In working together, children derive positive feelings from their ability to communicate, cooperate, negotiate, and problem solve. Most importantly, group play fosters a critical sense of belonging, which may compensate for negative feelings of isolation.

Planning a School-Age Program

The hospitalized school-age child can benefit from a Child Life program that is specifically designed for this age group. Child Life can foster age-appropriate developmental processes and provide a means of coping with stress, supplementing the school program, particularly during the summer months.

To reach the school-age child, a critical task is to provide appropriate materials in "an environment that will allow the child . . . to achieve independence from adults" (Lindheim et al., 1972, p. 58). The space must be welcoming to family, but most importantly, it must be child-centered to offer the children a sense of control, autonomy, security, and belonging. The space must provide enough room and flexibility to accommodate patients on gurneys and in wheelchairs.

In considering the developmental needs of school-age children, separate work areas must be provided so that several individuals can play cooperatively. In this way, many different activities may occur within the same multipurpose space, allowing children to make choices and work in preferred groups, usually determined by gender. In addition to large open areas for group play, the facility should include an expanded art center so that children may exercise fine motor skills through a variety of media. Access to a sink and stove are also beneficial for group cooking projects. Because the school-age child has developed an interest in the end-product of the work, plenty of table space may allow projects to be saved and left out until completion. The school-age child's cognitive level and increasing interest in learning will necessitate a variety of books, writing materials, scientific instruments, advanced medical equipment, and realistic props for dramatic play. Further, providing ample storage areas that are accessible by children for various materials helps promote their independence (Lindheim et al., 1972).

A Summertime School-Age Program

With the design of a space in mind, I was challenged to find an available room within the hospital to set up a summertime school-age program. The Teen Lounge became a hopeful prospect. Although not ideal in size and lacking natural light, the lounge would suffice with good organization and creative planning.

My goal was to make the space a multipurpose activity area that accommodated group play and created an atmosphere that was warm, pleasant, and age appropriate. I recruited four or five school-age children who were interested in making decorations to personalize the space. I followed their lead in designing the room and listened carefully to their suggestions of various activities of interest. I wanted to promote their competence, initiative, and independence by offering them the responsibility of creating a room that was all their own. Together, we set up three separate spaces (two round tables with several chairs and an open floor space) as well as a corkboard to display their artwork. Within a week the former Teen Lounge was transformed into a brightly colored "School-Age Activity Room," complete with a sign on the door.

Next I attempted to find the equipment and supplies necessary for various school-age activities and store them properly in the cupboards so they were easily accessible to the children. I organized the materials according to the kinds of play and projects the children were likely to engage in.

Dramatic and Medical Play

Through play acting the child releases fears, frustrations, and anxieties and is provided with the opportunity to reenact painful experiences repeatedly as a way of mastering the traumatic events. Materials for medical play and preparation include alcohol wipes, adhesive bandages, dolls, dress-up clothes, hair-dressing equipment, house keeping and kitchen props, IV lines, lengths of material, miniature wooden models of hospital equipment, puppets, syringes, stethoscopes, surgical masks, telephones, wigs, and the like.

Reading, Writing, and Story Telling

Children enjoy working on school-related skills and these enhance competence and sense of control. The room should be stocked with many diverse, developmentally appropriate books and magazines as well as paper and writing utensils. The children are encouraged to write letters to family and friends, compose a short story, make a hospital book, and keep a journal of their experiences. Reading and group storytelling can promote discussion of various topics related to the children's hospitalization. Similarly, writing is an effective means for the children to express feelings and reveal concerns to others. Publishing a newspaper can involve many children in drawing, writing, interviewing, reporting, copying, stapling, and distributing. By voicing opinions through written expression, the children may gain a heightened sense of accomplishment, mastery, and control over their hospital experience (Azarnoff & Flegal, 1975).

Constructive Play

School-age children enjoy exercising dexterity, creativity, problem-solving ability, and strength in building and manipulating materials (Azarnoff & Flegal, 1975). Equipment for making things may include glue, hammers, Legos, model-making kits, nails, origami, papier-mâché, train sets, scissors, sewing materials, string, yarn, various scraps for collage and woodwork, and the like.

Science Materials

To accommodate and promote the children's interest in learning and discovery, materials should include kaleidoscopes, magnets, newspapers, rulers, scales, science kits, tape measures, and the like.

Arts and Crafts

Creative expression through art has unlimited benefits for the school-age child. Not only is art a powerful means of self-expression, but it also enhances the child's feelings of control and mastery. Group art projects are also a valuable

source of social interaction. Supplies should include
brushes, clay, colored construction paper, pastels, glue,
paints, paper, play dough, markers, scissors, and odds and
ends of wood, paper, and material.

Games

Group games help children with organization, rules, compe-
tition, and cooperation. Popular games include bingo,
checkers, Clue, dominoes, Fooz-ball, Lotto, Memory, Monopoly, musical chairs, Nintendo, playing cards, puzzles,
Sorry, Trouble, and Uno.

Pets and Plants

Pets such as fish and guinea pigs give children the opportunity to be affectionate and to assume responsibility for their
care. Moreover, "animals have natural appeal for every child
for they have life, movement, surprise, and noise. They are
reassuring in a mechanical environment, nonthreatening,
and nothing is required of the child to enjoy them" (Azarnoff & Flegal, 1975, pp. 76–77).

Seeds, plants, and bulbs can be grown on the ward. They
provide opportunities for learning about the natural sciences and are a connection to the outdoors. For hospitalized
children who require ongoing nursing care, pets and plants
provide opportunities to show tenderness and care for
others.

Music

Music universally affects children. School-age children enjoy
listening to tapes, music making, and sing-alongs. Useful instruments include recorders, cymbals, drums, harmonicas,

triangles, chime bells, and maracas (Harvey & Hales-Tooke, 1972). Further, large cans, cartons, and blocks of wood are wonderful makeshift instruments that children can decorate and take home. Exploration with music encourages group discussion about many of the unfamiliar sounds that children hear in the hospital, such as the constant beeps from IV's and monitoring devices.

Special Events

The hospital virtually becomes a second home for many chronically ill children. Unfortunately, sickness occurs during holidays and birthdays. The "School-Age Activity Room" provides an appropriate space for acknowledging special occasions. Children can make decorations, plan activities, and celebrate birthdays. Organizing special events offers children an opportunity to assume responsibility, gain a sense of control, and interact within a social setting. Similarly, weekly scheduled cooking projects can promote cooperative efforts among children, group cohesiveness, and feelings of belonging.

Evaluating the Program

During previous summers, school-age children who participated in Child Life were intermixed with toddlers and preschool children in the main playroom. By creating a separate space for school-age children to play this summer, it became apparent that many school-age behaviors had been buffered by the mixed-age environment.

I witnessed the value of having a "School-Age Activity Room" as I watched the children involved in many age-appropriate behaviors and "normalizing" childhood experiences. Among school-age girls, a "girls only" club developed. The girls often became deeply involved in group medical play in which they organized medical props and role-played various hospital procedures. The girls also seemed to spend more time than the boys working individually on long-term art projects.

Among school-age boys, I observed a high frequency of social interaction and participation as well as increased competitive and aggressive behaviors. Some seemed to enjoy working with manipulatives and craft materials; others participated in active play. My observations led me to believe that the boys particularly needed appropriate outlets for strong feelings about being confined to the hospital, experiencing multiple invasive procedures, and being isolated from friends and family. Perhaps more materials for punching, throwing, beating, hammering, and pushing in addition to organized trips outdoors would have been beneficial.

One relationship developed between two "rehab" children that fully indicated the value of the program. Rocky, age 10, had been hospitalized for several months since an accident and had regained most of his daily functions including walking. Clyde, age 8, was in the initial stages of "rehab" and not yet able to walk, control his bowels, or speak without difficulty. Rocky and Clyde developed a turbulent yet special friendship in which they enjoyed each other's presence and collaborated in a variety of activities. Clyde admired Rocky who served as a role-model, offering Clyde hope and guidance. Rocky also experienced enjoyment, pride, and satisfaction in caring for Clyde tenderly and at times derisively. Clearly the support children give each other operates in reciprocal directions (Plank, 1971).The developmentally older child may function as a guide and protector of a developmentally younger child while gaining self-confidence for leadership efforts.

Conclusion

Many observations confirmed the importance of a play space within the hospital for school-age children, especially during the summer months. During the school year, this age group attends a school program that addresses their developmental tasks. Since school-age children are particularly concerned with control, competence, and acceptance among peers, they need a social space and the appropriate tools to master age-appropriate challenges. Group play within the hospital is "a vehicle through which the school-age child explores potential friendships and solidifies bonds" (Thompson & Stanford, 1981, p. 73). By facilitating a critical sense of belonging, children are better able to cope with the stresses imposed by illness and hospitalization, and thus potentials for development, learning, and mastery are maximized. Clearly, the peer group is a critical focus for development at this stage.

By the end of the summer "The School-Age Activity Room" was a space conducive to productive play experiences for children 6 to 12 years of age. These children previously may have "fallen through the cracks" by Child Life.

References

Azarnoff, P., & Flegal, S. (1975). *A pediatric play program.* Springfield, IL: Charles C. Thomas.

Eckenhoff, J. E. (1953). Relationship of anesthesia to postoperative personality changes in children. *American Journal of Disabled Children, 86,* 587–591.

Harvey, S., & Hales-Tooke, A. (1972). *Play in hospital.* London: Faber & Faber.

James, F. E. (1960). Behavior reactions of normal children to common operations. *Practitioner, 185,* 339–342.

Lindheim, R., Glaser, H., & Coffin, C. (1972). *Changing hospital environments for children.* Cambridge, MA: Harvard University Press.

Piaget, J., & Inhelder, B. (1969). *The psychology of the child.* New York: Basic Books.

Plank, E. (1971). *Working with children in hospitals* (2nd ed.). Cleveland: Press of Case Western Reserve University.

Thompson, R. H., & Stanford, G. (1981). *Child Life in hospitals.* Springfield, IL: Charles C. Thomas.

Part Six

The Nonhospital Setting

14

Child Life
in a Nonhospital Setting

A Play Group
for Substance Abusers
and Their Drug-Exposed
Infants and Toddlers

LAUREN MANHEIMER

Chemical Addiction Recovery Efforts (CARE) at Children's Hospital, Oakland, California, is a model infant–parent program that serves children from birth to age 3, who have been exposed to drugs in utero, and their chemically dependent mothers. The Center has three primary goals: (1) to facilitate the mother's recovery from addictive disease; (2) to aid the development of the affected infants and toddlers; (3) to assist in keeping mother and babies together and decrease foster care placement.

The CARE Center uses a family-centered approach as the primary modality for serving children with special needs (Dunst, Trivette, & Deal, 1988; Johnson, McGonigel, & Kaufman, 1989; McGonigel & Garland, 1988; Shelton, Jeppson, & Johnson, 1987). Experience suggests that children born with a biological insult such as drug and/or alcohol exposure in utero can develop optimally in a supportive caretaking environment (Samaroff & Chandler, 1975; Samaroff & Fiese, 1990). The more vulnerable the child, the more critical is the quality of caretaking in determining developmental outcomes.

The Mothers in CARE

Chemically dependent women live in a society that rejects them and frequently blames them for their addiction, increasing their sense of failure and inadequacy before motherhood has even begun (St. Claire & Berkowitz, 1994). Because at CARE the caretakers are the essential element in any child's environment, the mothers are the primary focus for intervention services. Although the extended family may be involved, the model is intended to serve three clients: the mother, the child, and the relationship between them (St. Claire & Berkowitz, 1994). Enhancing the birth mother's self-esteem, parenting skills, and attachment relationship offers the potential for the mother to provide successfully for her baby, even in the face of addictive disease.

The mothers in CARE are ages 18 to 25. Most of these young women live in poverty, have a dual diagnosis, and have partners who are either abusive or no longer involved with them and their children. At present, three of the women have more than one child.

Clearly, the recovering mothers have difficulties in their lives, past and present, which interfere with their ability to relate to their children. Many of the women's mothers, themselves often young adolescents when they became pregnant, were substance abusers, and the younger generation of mothers have strong anger and feelings of failure and abandonment by their own mothers. The mothers' childhoods were characterized by abuse and neglect.

The mothers often feel guilty about having used drugs during their pregnancy and fear they cannot meet their infants' needs. They often have unrealistic expectations for their new child and harbor anger toward the infant, who frequently was conceived unexpectedly in their already chaotic lives.

The mother's psychological distress with regard to the birth, her unconscious conflicts related to her childhood experience, and the frequent separations due to the infant's illnesses contribute to difficulties in the relationship between the infant and mother. However, despite the difficulties, the special bond between mother and child if supported can help the mother's recovery process by enhancing her overall investment in her child, thereby fostering feelings of worth and adequacy. For many chemically dependent women, parenthood is one of the few socially acceptable means of self-esteem available to them (Rosenbaum, 1981).

The Children in CARE

The young children at the CARE Center are often drug-exposed in utero with potentially a variety of deleterious effects on their overall health and development. Many of these infants are born prematurely and remain medically fragile throughout infancy and later. A premature arrival of the infant may occur before the mother has consolidated her feelings about the new infant or has developed a sense of psychological readiness. The mother has likely not had a positive birthing experience and must deal with feelings of failure and grief over the loss of the fantasy baby she failed to deliver (Brazelton, 1982; Klaus & Kennell, 1976).

In general, preterm infants tend to be less active and alert than full-term infants, making fewer responses and demands of their mothers. The children frequently show developmental difficulties ranging from significant global delays to fairly specific delays that may take years to identify and assess.

Also, mothers of preterms are less actively involved with their babies. They make less body contact (DiVitto & Goldberg, 1979; Klaus, Kennell, Plumb, & Zuehlke, 1970; Leifer, Leiderman, Barnett, & Williams, 1972), spend less time face to face (Klaus et al., 1970), smile at their infants less (Leifer et al., 1972), touch them less (DiVitto & Goldberg, 1979; Klaus et al., 1970; Leifer et al., 1972), and talk to them less (DiVitto & Goldberg, 1979). Drug-exposed infants may also manifest behavioral difficulties such as irregular sleep–wake patterns, attention deficit disorder, temper tantrums, distractibility, and irritability.

Clearly, prematurity and prenatal drug exposure interrupt the development of interactive skills in both mother and infant, hindering the development of a secure attachment relationship (Goldberg, 1982). The major realistic concerns about the infant's health and the usually protracted period of hospitalization following the birth interfere with early opportunities for bonding (Goldberg, 1982).

The CARE Program

The Center offers a wide array of interdisciplinary support services, both center based and home based, that are individually geared to infant–mother needs. Contact with the Center enables the clients to participate actively in the program, obtain nutritional meals, live a healthy life, and maintain a safe home environment. Among the concrete resources offered are transportation services, emergency food, infant formula, diapers, and advocacy with bureaucratic systems.

The team that delivers these services is comprised of three infant development specialists, a clinical nurse specialist, an occupational therapist, a drug and alcohol counselor, a child care worker, a psychologist, a psychiatrist, and a pediatrician. Although each family has a single primary therapist, the team reviews cases and consults during weekly scheduled sessions. The Center acknowledges that "the woman's need for recovery and parenting support and the infant's ongoing medical and developmental needs must be addressed simultaneously and in the context of the relationship between mother and child" (St. Claire & Berkowitz, 1994, p. 126; Pawl, 1993). The Center recognizes that women struggling with addictive disease need the support of other recovering women to help them manage feelings appropriately, build self-esteem, and feel accepted and understood (St. Claire & Berkowitz, 1994).

The family's problems are addressed through a combination of services. These services include chemical dependency education, relapse prevention groups, on-site Narcotics Anonymous (NA) meetings, home visits with one-to-one counseling, and referrals to residential treatment. These recovery services support the mother's transition to a "clean" and sober state and attempt to shift her attention from maintaining her addiction to her parenting responsibilities.

The mother's investment in her child is enhanced by offering developmental guidance, education and information, parenting support groups, and infant–parent psychotherapy. Infant–parent psychotherapy as developed by Selma Fraiberg is the primary approach used by the Center (Fraiberg, Adelson, & Shapiro, 1975). This method focuses on the infant's needs and on the mother's unconscious conflicts that are associated with traumatic childhood. Infant–parent psychotherapy involves continuous observation of the infant in the natural home setting and a tactful, nondidactic education of the mother in recognition of her baby's needs and

signals (Fraiberg, Adelson, & Shapiro, 1976). Through exploration of the mother's experiences of emotional neglect
as a child and her ambivalence toward her infant, the mother
may gain critical insight, which may help her avoid reen-
acting her own childhood conflicts and strengthen her relationship with her child.

The services provided for children are designed to promote their health, growth, development, and psychological
well-being. They include pediatric care, developmental assessments, early intervention home guidance, and the therapeutic nursery. The nursery program offers daily respite
care for the mothers and a variety of activities to assess and
meet the developmental needs of the children in a warm,
safe, and consistent environment. The activities are designed
to develop gross motor and fine motor skills, language, sen-
sorimotor perception, and behavioral organization. The program supports diversity, respect for others, self-awareness,
and self-esteem. By observing and assessing the children's
developmental progress in the nursery, child care workers
provide valuable information for the therapists. The nursery
reinforces the importance of the family unit of mother and
child by encouraging the mother's involvement in play with
her child and sensitive separation and reunion rituals.

Play in the Center

I noted that typically mothers arrived at the Center in a
harried state, literally dropping off their children in the nursery, and scurrying away to appointments. Whenever I invited
mothers to play with their children, suggesting that it would
help create a smoother transition to the nursery environment, the mothers resisted the opportunity, finding time
only to sign in their children and quickly turn away. Curi-
ously, the children seldom protested.

When a child arrived at the nursery distressed, at times I
requested that the mother remain with her child until he or

she was comforted and able to engage in play. During one incident, the mother was overtly flustered by my request. She pulled her $1^1/_2$-year-old son by the arm to the bean bag chair in the corner of the nursery. Hastily, she plopped him down and stuck a bottle into his mouth. The mother rolled up a blanket and placed it beneath her son's chin to prop up the bottle. The child sucked on his bottle, his body tense, his stare cold and blank. His muffled cry persisted. With no tender caress, words of comfort, or attempts to play, the mother darted toward the door and told me, "He'll fall asleep eventually."

Many observations such as the preceding suggested a lack of success in fostering the mothers' involvement in play experiences with their children. Repeatedly I observed separation rituals that lacked warmth and sensitivity and reunions without the hint of delight. I seldom saw mothers play with their children or playfully hold and stroke them. Rare was the tender gaze into the children's eyes. Mostly I observed harsh interactions with anger, frustration, and chaos. Clearly the Center could benefit from paying increased attention to its "third client," that is, the relationship between the mother and child, particularly the role of play in the mother–child interaction.

I noted that many of the women who resisted play with their children were at a point in their recovery where there was a sense of urgency about themselves and their needs. When these mothers arrived at the Center, they rushed to scheduled activities and appointments. Finding time for a slow good-bye or playing with the children to foster a smooth transition was difficult for these mothers who already were overwhelmed by the grave circumstances of their lives. Many are adolescents, developmentally delayed, depressed, battered, homeless, hungry, and generally deprived. These women find little room for their children in their chaotic lives. The mothers, as are the children, are overtly starved for loving attention from their mothers. The mothers have come to value the Center as their sanctuary where they feel safe, nurtured, and supported without judgment. The mothers cherish their time in group treatment as a needed respite from their children, who are being cared for in the nursery.

A Play Group at CARE

At the Center, I attempted to see if the mother–child relationship could be strengthened by promoting play between these young mothers and their infants and toddlers. For many of these women, the concept of play is utterly foreign. Many tell of their lack of play as children. Frequently they themselves had caregivers who were neglectful and abusive.

In coordination with one of the Center's infant development specialists, I developed a play group that meets one hour each week. The group is comprised of recovering mothers and their infants and toddlers. It is led by two facilitators from the Center's nursery. The goals are threefold:

1. Promotion of the mother–child attachment relationship by focusing on communication through play.
2. Promotion of the child's social–emotional, cognitive, and motor development through playful interactions that emphasize social reciprocity, exploration, and movement.
3. Support of the mother's recovery and development of self-esteem by expanding her modes of expression with her child.

The Center's nursery is the most suitable location to hold the play group. An ideal size, the nursery is bright and the furnishings are child-scaled. The space imparts feelings of warmth, fun, and youth. With its soft carpet and natural light, the room provides an unspoken invitation to play.

All of the mothers and children are already familiar with the nursery and associate the space with play. In preparing the nursery for the play group, all the chairs are removed to encourage the mothers to sit on the rug with their children. Mother and child therefore are interacting on the same level.

Fliers announcing the time, location, place, and description of the group are decorated by some of the Center's children and are posted throughout the Center. Copies also are given to the therapists, case managers, and child care staff, who in turn distribute them to their clients with verbal encouragement to attend.

The activities engage the mothers and infants and toddlers in relaxing, creative, and playful endeavors. By demonstrating various developmentally appropriate activities for mothers to use in playfully engaging with their infants and toddlers, we hope that the mothers may increase their enjoyment of mothering experiences. Surprisingly the activities facilitate the mothers' own conversations regarding their memories of play as children. Many report never having had any play experiences or toys.

The Play Group Program

Rug Time

1. "Check in";
2. Songs, movement, finger play;
3. Introduction of day's activity.

When the mothers and their infants and toddlers arrive for the play group, they are asked to join in a circle on the carpet—"rug time." Each mother is asked to "check in" for herself and for her child. The process of "checking in" is one with which the women are familiar in that it begins all of their therapy groups. The mothers are asked to introduce themselves and briefly describe how they are feeling. In "checking in" for their infants and toddlers, the mothers are encouraged to interpret their children's cues, assess their needs, and gain awareness of their emotional states.

Following "check in" are a few songs that involve movement and finger play. These exercises effectively engage the group and promote the children's language and motor development.

Activities

1. Sensory exploration: bubbles, "flubber," water play, and mirror play;
2. Food preparation, feeding;
3. Manipulatives: rattle tracking, reaching, "bait casting," and block activities;
4. Games: language games (copy cat), searching games (peek-a-boo, hide-and-seek, "guess where"), space games (stacking and "fill'er up"), sorting games, and simple puzzles;
5. Art projects: napkin dyeing, rattle making, hand prints, and finger painting.

After introducing the day's activity, the necessary materials are presented to the group. The various activities are designed to engage the participants in playful interactions in which mother and children feel challenged and triumphant. The mothers are encouraged to show warmth, love, and pride in their children's achievements without demanding success (Gordon, 1970).

Games involving stacking, searching, filling, and dumping blocks enhance the child's physical dexterity, effectively promoting a sense of space relations. Moreover, exercises in imitative dialogue between mother and infant exercise sound-making and language development.

Peek-a-boo and hide-and-seek games foster object constancy and add to the child's understanding that the world has dependability and order (Kleeman, 1967; J. Oremland, 1973). Object constancy, the capacity to maintain an internalized representation of the mother when she is not physically present, allows the child to separate from the mother.

Food preparation as a group activity is facilitated, and the mothers are encouraged to hold, smile, and talk to their infants and toddlers while feeding them.

Although the activities promote the child's cognitive, physical, social, and psychological development, additional purposes are served. For example, rattle games foster the coordination of the infant's senses (seeing and hearing) with ability to move (tracking, grasping, and searching). However, rattle making is also a creative endeavor yielding a concrete toy that can be taken home, enriching the children's home environment.

Art Review and Rug Time

Each play group session ends with a "rug time" circle. The mothers and infants and toddlers return to the rug and are given the opportunity to share observations and present their "work." The play group closes with cookies and a song. The CARE staff and I believe that ending the group as it began conveys a sense of wholeness and completion.

Discussion

The play group program evolved more slowly than anticipated. Engaging these women in groups is difficult, especially when the group is new and unfamiliar. Lack of trust in authority, including the health care system, is pervasive in this population. Recruitment to and maintenance of attendance requires frequent reminders, advertising, and most importantly, patience. It is critical to be flexible, yet be able to convey to the young mothers the firm belief that consistent attendance is a crucial ingredient for effectiveness.

Another problem arose from the attempt to limit the play group to infants and toddlers. In general, it is easier to foster playful and sensitive interaction in a group of mothers with infants and toddlers than if the age range of the children is broader. Several mothers expressed difficulties in finding child care for their older children. At first, the mothers were allowed to bring all of their children to the play group. However, the environment quickly became chaotic. To hold a successful play group session it became necessary for the Center to provide child care for older siblings during the play group hour.

Another difficulty arose from not fully anticipating the mothers' responses to the experience. As the mothers became involved in the play group activities, it also became difficult for them to interact with their infants and toddlers because of activation of their own extraordinary neediness. Their play quickly became intense, almost frantic manifestations of personal yearning and regressive behaviors. They became needy, demanding sympathy and comforting. Often they wanted to be fed. In trying to persuade them to play with their infants and toddlers, I often asked, "What is your baby doing right now?" The response frequently was, "Look at what *I'm* doing right now."

During one play group session, I organized a napkin dyeing activity in which the mothers and infants and toddlers placed droppers full of food coloring onto folded sheets resulting in symmetrical designs. Many of the women commented that they could not believe that they could create something that beautiful. With great urgency each of the women completed several patterns, but their involvement with their infants and toddlers was minimal. I noticed that one mother froze in the middle of her play, holding a curious stare. I asked if she wanted to share her thoughts with the group. She revealed sadly, "When I was a child, I didn't play at all. I saw my sister get shot. I grew up fast." In those few piercing words, it was apparent that she was reexperiencing sadness and loss that she carries into her motherhood. Within several minutes she picked up her child and held him against her breast, playing with him with tenderness and sensitivity.

Some of the women were able to verbalize that they felt overwhelmed by the temptation of drugs and the chaos in their lives, and that those feelings interfered with their ability to play with their children and to tolerate their children's playful behaviors. One poignant discussion was initiated by a mother who was struggling with her exploratory, danger-prone toddler. Her interactions with her daughter were largely negative—a sea of "no's." She sensed that she constantly and fearfully restricted her child's every activity. Sadly she added, "She limits me, too."

The woman expressed memories of harsh and abusive "no's" from her mother, sensing that she had internalized her mother's negative and oppressive "no's." Her understanding that "no" was important for safety was intertwined with her understanding that "no" was also an expression of anger, frustration, and a way of being abusive. Her memories led to a group discussion about toddlerhood, firm boundaries, and how limits also could be expressions of love. At that point one woman asked me, "Could I bring my other son to the play group next week? I want to have special time with him, too, and show him that I love him."

One time in a play group session, we showed a video about speaking in rhyme that presented songs, finger games, and lullabies of different cultures around the world. The video beautifully portrayed sensitive interactions between adults and children. While we watched the video, I encouraged the mothers to hold, rock, and feed their infants and toddlers. The mothers expressed their delight in the experience and shared many childhood memories. One mother revealed sadly, "I don't think that anyone sang lullabies to me as a child. When it was bedtime, someone just put me in a crib and went on to attend to the other nine."

When the video ended, the group discussed the value of rhyme and song. One African-American woman said, "I guess songs are important because they remind you of who you are and where you come from. They can make you feel a part of something. They can be passed on to your children. I want to learn more African songs and dances."

In the play group, we encouraged the women to share stories, songs, rhymes and dance with their infants and toddlers. Such forms of play are shown as effective means of communicating and solidifying the unique bond between mother and child.

Summary

In researching, designing, and implementing the play group, it is clear that Child Life can have an important place in nonhospital, community-based organizations such as the CARE Center. My knowledge of child development, the needs of families at risk, and the Child Life techniques of therapeutic play with highly vulnerable families have been critical to my ability and confidence to carry out my play group project. The project has led me to considerations I never anticipated.

At the Center, developmental progress by the children and the mothers is palpable. The play group has become a critical component of its program. In addition to the developmental benefits of the play activities themselves, the play group helps the mother to recognize that mother–child play is a way of conveying to the children a sense of the mother's dependability, devotion, sensitivity, and flexibility. The play group emphasizes that play is a manifestation of the loving attachment that enhances the infant's and toddler's ability to form relationships throughout life (Gordon, 1970). Although the initial play group sessions emphasized the mothers' needs, the group slowly and increasingly has focused on the developmental needs of the infants and toddlers and the mother–child relationship itself. As the mothers express their feelings, they increasingly develop an ability to play with their children.

In participating in play with their infants and toddlers, the mothers experience rewards and develop positive attitudes toward exploratory play behaviors. The pleasure derived from the play potentially enhances the mothers' self-esteem and promotes play experiences outside the group.

It is my hope that all of the mothers at the Center will one day cherish the beautiful and special smiles that their children reserve only for them during play and other caring activities. At that point, the attachment relationship has been effectively strengthened.

References

Brazelton, T. (1982). Behavioral assessment of the premature infant: Uses in intervention. In M. Klaus & M. Robertson (Eds.), *Birth, interaction and attachment* (pp. 85–92). Skillman, NJ: Johnson & Johnson Baby Products, Co.

DiVitto, B., & Goldberg, S. (1979). The development of early parent–infant interaction as a function of newborn medical status. In T. Field, A. Sostek, S. Goldberg, & H. Shuman (Eds.), *Infants born at risk* (pp. 311–332). Holliswood, NY: Spectrum.

Dunst, C., Trivette, C., & Deal, A. (1988). *Enabling and empowering families: Principles and guidelines for practice.* Cambridge, MA: Brookline Books.

Fraiberg, S., Adelson, E., & Shapiro, V. (1975). Ghosts in the nursery: A psychoanalytic approach to the problems of impaired infant–mother relationships. *Journal of the American Academy of Child Psychiatry, 14,* 387–421.

Fraiberg, S., Adelson, E., & Shapiro, V. (1976). Infant–parent psychotherapy on behalf of a child in a critical nutritional state. *The Psychoanalytic Study of the Child, 31,* 461–491. New Haven, CT: Yale University Press.

Goldberg, S. (1982). Prematurity: Effects on parent–infant interaction. In J. Belsky (Ed.), *In the beginning: Readings on infancy.* New York: Columbia University Press.

Gordon, I. (1970). *Baby learning through baby play.* New York: St. Martin's Press.

Gordon, I. (1971). *On early learning.* Washington, DC: Association for Supervision and Curriculum Development.

Johnson, B., McGonigel, M., & Kaufman, R. (1989). *Guidelines and recommended practices for the individualized family service plan.* Washington, DC: Association for the Care of Children's Health.

Klaus, M., & Kennell, J. (1976). *Maternal–infant bonding.* St. Louis: C. V. Mosby.

Klaus, M., Kennell, J., Plumb, N., & Zuehlke, S. (1970). Human maternal behavior at the first contact with her young. *Pediatrics, 46,* 187–192.

Kleeman, J. (1967). The peek-a-boo game. *The Psychoanalytic Study of the Child, 22,* 239–252. New York: International Universities Press.

Leifer, A., Leiderman, P., Barnett, C., & Williams, J. (1972). Effects of mother–infant separation on maternal attachment behavior. *Child Development, 43,* 1203–1218.

McGonigel, M., & Garland, C. (1988). The individualized family service plan and the early intervention team: Team and family issues and recommended practices. *Infants and Young Children, 1,* 10–21.

Oremland, J. (1973). The jinx game. *The Psychoanalytic Study of the Child, 28,* 419–431. New Haven, CT: Yale University Press.

Pawl, J. (1993). Interventions to strengthen relationships between infants and drug abusing or recovering parents. *Zero to Three, August/September,* 6–10.

Rosenbaum, M. (1981). *Women on heroin.* New Brunswick, NJ: Rutgers University Press.

Samaroff, A., & Chandler, M. (1975). Reproductive risk and the continuum of caretaking casualty. In F. Horowitz, M.

Hetherington, S. Scarr-Salapatek, & G. Siegel (Eds.), *Review of child development research* (Vol. 4), pp. 187–244. Chicago: University of Chicago Press.

Samaroff, A., & Fiese, B. (1990). Transaction regulation and early intervention. In S. Meisels & J. Shankoff (Eds.), *Handbook of early childhood intervention* (pp. 119–149). New York: Cambridge University Press.

Shelton, T., Jeppson, E., & Johnson, B. (1987). *Family-centered care for children with special health care needs.* Washington, DC: Association for the Care of Children's Health.

St. Claire, N., & Berkowitz, G. (1994). Reaching the child through the family. In C. Puttkammer (Ed.), *Working with substance-exposed children.* Tucson, AZ: Therapy Skill Builders.

Part Seven

A Developmental Model

15

A Developmental Model for Training Child Life Infant Specialists for Early Intervention Programs in Hospitals and Group Care Settings

EVELYN K. OREMLAND, JANE BOWYER,
JOAN C. HENRY, STEPHANIE ERNST, CAROL GEORGE,
BETH SAMELS, and ANN COPENHAGEN

In the United States, two-thirds of all hospitalized children under age 15 are younger than 4 years of age. One-half of these children, exclusive of physically well newborns, are in their first year of life (National Center for Health Statistics, 1992). This population includes fragile, prematurely born infants, drug-exposed and AIDS-infected infants and toddlers, and young children with various developmental delays. These at-risk children benefit from their medically trained caregivers and from nonmedical personnel who are trained in child development and other psychosocial approaches. These nonmedically trained professionals include psychologists, social workers, and a growing field of professionals called Child Life Specialists (Gaynard, 1990).

Child Life Specialists focus on child development as it is affected by illness and hospitalization (Brazelton & Thompson, 1988). Generally centered in play programs for pediatric hospital care, Child Life Specialists enable children to play while they are hospitalized to enhance normal growth and development. These specialists help children prepare for medical procedures via developmentally appropriate play to assist them in making sense of their frequently bewildering and painful experiences. The goals of the specialty are to minimize the potential traumas of childhood illness and hospitalization while supporting children's normal developmental progressions.

Child Life Specialists provide supportive relationships for parents of sick children in their caregiving roles and child development education for pediatric staff to enhance their interactions with children. An international body, The Child Life Council, defines the professional roles and standards for the Child Life field.

The education and training for this field are specialized yet grounded in normative development and experiences with "normal" infants. The Child Life Program at Mills College, Oakland, California, has been a model for the field for 20 years. This rigorous, research-based training program provides students with course work and field experiences that prepare them for work with children in hospitals.

The Mills College Child Life Program began to emphasize work with infants following the growing body of research on the vulnerabilities of sick and hospitalized infants and of ameliorative interventions. Few training programs currently prepare nonmedical caregivers for work with the infant population.

Two fundamental constructs have guided the development of the Child Life Program design: identification of the necessary bodies of knowledge and reflection and the ongoing process of finding meanings and connections in theory and practice (Richert, 1989; Schulman, 1987). Together these constructs underlie simultaneous study of theories and practical applications. Child Life students need subject knowledge in child development, children's responses to crises, and methodology for appropriate interventions with children in medical settings. Journal writing and daily "debriefings" are practiced in the hospital setting and in the infant–toddler laboratory settings to encourage student reflection and evaluation of theories in conjunction with practice. Informal classroom seminar discussions extend the collegial environment for this practice, as established early in the student's 2-year master's degree program by a retreat on the infant attended by faculty and Child Life students.

The program described for training infant specialists, chiefly for master's degree candidates with the Child Life emphasis, integrates practical experiences in the hospital and infant care settings with course work in child development and childhood illness phenomena. Field experiences in normative and special areas, and study of salient theories in each, are concurrent, integrated through reflective thinking in seminars and "debriefings." A conceptualization of this professional training model is depicted in Figure 15.1.

The Infant–Toddler Laboratory School Experience

The Child Life curriculum is integrally related to the early childhood education program in which the laboratory school associated with the education department provides an in-house group setting for young children's care and learning. The infant–toddler component introduced in 1991

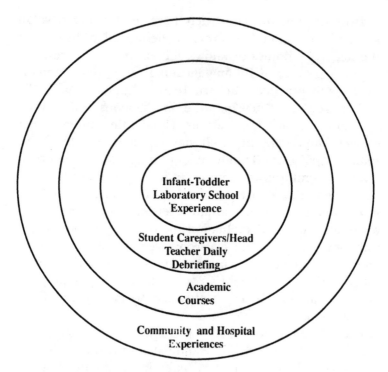

Figure 15.1 Design for Professional Education and Training Child Life / Infant Care Model

specifically to support the Child Life Specialty provides students with first-hand knowledge and understanding of normal infant development. Students spend a semester of the 2-year program in this setting, integrating theory and practice through simultaneous analyses and reflection.

The Mills College Infant–Toddler Program

Eleven infants, ages 3 to 36 months, form the nucleus of the infant–toddler program. The program operates 5 days a week from 9:00 a.m. to 11:30 a.m., with an extended care option available until 5:15 p.m. to accommodate working parents. The head teacher and a team of Mills College graduate students in education are the caregivers for four to five mornings per week. The ratio of caregivers to infants is generally one adult to two or three children.

Observation of and interaction with the children and their parents enable the study of behavior, the development of relationships, developmental progression, individual differences, and how children learn. Strategies for interactions with children evolve from recognizing children's feelings and needs and acquiring a sensitivity to the pace set by each child. Concurrent communication with parents ensures a supportive process relative to each child's care at home and in the school. Rather than illustrating "how to" techniques, the emphasis is on implementation of ideas.

The Head Teacher

The head teacher, an infant development practitioner and early childhood educator, fulfills an important role in this program. Her multifaceted responsibilities include planning, implementing, and maintaining a developmentally appropriate program for infants and toddlers (Honig & Lally, 1981; Torelli, 1989). She orchestrates relationships with parents and children, sets a conducive environment, models appropriate practice, and supervises, trains, and evaluates the student teachers.

To establish optimal communication with parents and to achieve effective integration with family care, the head teacher visits each child's home at the outset of the new semester. Knowing the infants in their environment and developing a working relationship with parents are the major goals of the initial visit.

The Students

Philosophically, respect for each child is critical (Gerber, 1984). The students as caregivers pay careful attention to each child's cues and respond accordingly. Rather than viewing care as a series of tasks, the student actively involves the infant in the caregiving processes and in the surrounding world, as noted in the following student journal:

> At the far end of the room, in the diaper-changing area, Nora is changing 6-month-old Sandra's diaper. Nora carefully lays Sandra on the mat, talking to Sandra about what she is doing and giving Sandra an opportunity to take in the environment. Nora removes Sandra's jumper and changes the diaper. Sandra and Nora mutually respond by eye contact. Nora imitates some of Sandra's babbles and tells her that she is going to pick her up and return her to the infant area.

Primary caregivers are "assigned" to nurture trust; that is, a primary caregiver is consistently responsible for a particular child every day and for daily recording of infant–caregiver interactions to facilitate the ongoing relationship with parents (Bowlby, 1982). Often the primary relationship between the caregiver and child is initiated spontaneously by the child. A caregiver, in the first days of care, will note that an infant has "chosen" her.

The primary caregiver supplements the parent's role. From the role of subsidiary caregiver, a "curriculum" for the infants evolves, during which each caregiver presents the opportunity for the child to explore, learn, and develop.

Jean Piaget (1952) identifies how these maturing interactions evolve (Almy, 1982). He describes that from experience beginning in infancy human beings construct their knowledge and build their changing views of the world as the following example from a student caregiver's journal demonstrates:

It is midmorning and four children are settled around the table snacking on melon cubes and cereal O's. Karen, a caregiver, is sitting with them. Twenty-month-old Melody pours her cereal from the cup to the table, carefully inspecting each piece. Eighteen-month-old Terry is fascinated with the top on his water cup and tries to find a way to remove it. Twenty-two-month-old Carol has her special bunny sitting with her at the table and is feeding cereal and sips of water to her bunny and herself. Thirteen-month-old Peter is taking in the scene. Karen reflects aloud what she sees while providing the children [with] the freedom to explore and learn from this everyday occurrence.

Throughout the semester each student is videotaped in the classroom. The tapes are viewed by the staff and fellow students so that the students may evaluate their practice, assess their progress, and reflect on their development in the teaching and caregiving process.

The Parents

In keeping with recent infant research, relationships between the infants and those important in their lives are stressed in the infant–toddler program (Axtman, 1984; Moss, 1993). The relationships with parents are acknowledged as key in initiating the transition to group care, especially during initial separations. Parents are encouraged to remain with their children for as many days as necessary until their children develop relationships with the caregivers. The staff discusses with the parents separation anxiety, attachment, and autonomy issues. With increased understanding, parents become more skillful in supporting their children through these developmental challenges (Miller, 1993).

Daily interactions between parents and caregivers occur when the child is brought to and picked up from school. Notes written each day by both parents and caregivers record caregiving information regarding the infant on a chart established for each. Sleeping, eating, diaper changes, the child's mood, and brief descriptions of the day are recorded.

Two parent–teacher conferences are scheduled each year, and activities to bring parents and caregivers together are held throughout the year. These meetings enable parents and caregivers to share observations and to address parents' issues and concerns. A brunch each semester is a focal point for staff–parent, parent–parent, and adult–child interactions in a supportive and informal environment. The fundamental message is that staff care is an extension of and not a substitute for parent care (Provence, 1989). Parents and teachers are in partnership.

Student Caregivers and Head Teacher Daily "Debriefing"

"Debriefing" meetings follow each day's session in which the head teacher and student caregivers discuss the children. Study of how theory clarifies practice and how practice clarifies theory integrates the laboratory and course work.

The daily evaluation meetings revolve around a variety of topics. As example:

> Four student teachers and the head teacher, while discussing the events of the morning, focus on a student's description of a difficulty that Teddy, $9^1/2$ months old, has in separating from his mother each morning. The student tells the staff that this difficulty has intensified in the last few days. It is noted that the mother appears distressed during the separations.
>
> The staff asks about Teddy's reactions, how long it takes the mother to say good-bye, and about the student's follow-up with the mother. Separation anxiety for infant and mother and its place in development become the topics of the discussion. Students share their ideas on making the morning departure smoother and how best to support Teddy and his mother.

Student Journals

Student teachers keep a journal of their classroom experiences. In the journal, students reflect on their experiences, ask questions, and discuss how course work readings influence their practice. The journal, rather than being a narrative of the day's events, is a chronicle of the student's growth and development. The head teacher responds to journal entries, creating a written dialogue with each student. These integrated studies and experiences of well children become the basis for work with infants in hospitals.

Academic Courses

Courses on Normative Development

Integral to the training program are related courses including "Theory and Practice of Early Childhood Education," "Research Methods for Observation of Young Children," "Developmental Learning (Cognitive Development)," and "History and Theories of Play" (Table 15.1). Each course has a component focusing on infants and toddlers. One course, "The Psychology of Infancy," is devoted exclusively to infant development, presenting research and theories that describe the behavior, thoughts, and feelings of infants. Normative development is emphasized, following current models of developmental psychopathology, which propose that training and intervention programs for all infant professionals, including those who work with atypical infants, be thoroughly grounded in normal development (Lewis & Miller, 1990). In addition, the "Infancy Course" describes infant development in the context of interconnected systems of social relationships and institutions—an ecological systems approach (Bronfenbrenner, 1979).

TABLE 15.1

Academic Courses (Focus on Infants) for
Child Life and Early Childhood Programs

Studies of Normative Development	Studies of Hospitalized Infants
Infancy	The Hospitalized Child
Research Methods for Observing Children	Field Experience and Seminar in Child Life (with hospital internship)
Theory and Practice of Early Childhood Education (with field practice, infant–toddler care)	Topics in Child Health
History and Theories of Play in Human Development, Culture, and Education	Medical Information for Work with Children in Hospitals
Development and Learning in Young Children	
Social and Emotional Development of Young Children	
Educational Role of the Family	
Attachment and Loss	

Students observe infants and toddlers in the Children's
School laboratory setting for physical–motor, perceptual,
cognitive, social, and emotional development. This experience vitalizes the otherwise abstract, intellectual concepts
and creates ecological links between the infant and his or
her family and group care. Detailed observations of infants
from the laboratory school are incorporated into the course
discussions and papers. Special seminars on attachment theory and a course on children with special needs are available.

Courses for Work with Infants in Hospitals

The specialized courses for the Child Life Program present
the theoretical contexts for understanding hospital experiences of children. The "Hospitalized Child" is the primary

course in which the initial study is on the responses of infants to hospitalization (Oremland & Oremland, 1973). Aspects of infant development challenged by hospitalization and illness are reviewed, including the salience of relationship, attachment, and separation issues (Goldberger, 1988; Provence, 1989). Classical studies in these areas, including those of René Spitz (1945), John Bowlby (1982), and Mary Ainsworth (Ainsworth, Blehar, Waters, & Wall, 1987), are discussed.

Following the work of George Engel and others (Engel & Reichsman, 1956; Goldberger & Wolfer, 1991; E. Oremland, 1990), illness and institutional experience as superimposed on the developmental challenges of infancy become the context for understanding infants and toddlers in the hospital. The play of these children and their play while hospitalized are studied, particularly referencing Erik Erikson's (1963) studies on the meanings of play.

In the course "Child Health Topics," prematurity and its effects on development and experience are studied (Goldberg, 1982; Gutkind, 1991; The Infant Health and Development Program, 1990). Staff, family, and patient interactions in Intensive Care nurseries (Gottwald & Thurman, 1990) and how decisions are made in these circumstances are reviewed (Guillemin & Holmstrom, 1986; Willis, 1991). Juxtaposed with these issues, the problematic situations of teenage motherhood in interface with infant development and work in hospitals are detailed (Hartley, White, & Yogman, 1989).

The field work seminar, generally taken for three semesters, enables students to discuss and analyze their interactions with children in hospitals, and it is in addition to regularly scheduled individual hospital supervisory conferences. This clinically oriented course meets weekly in conjunction with the students' participation in hospital field work. Student journals are studied and interactions are discussed among the students who work approximately 20 hours weekly as interns in the area's major hospitals and pediatric units. Differing influences in the various settings, often five to seven hospitals each semester, provide opportunities to study the manifestations of various impingements. A course in medical information taught by a pediatrician provides a basis for understanding the language of the hospital and of illness.

Community and Hospital Experiences

Infant Group Care in the Community

In order to provide students with broader perspectives on children's group care beyond what the college laboratory settings offer, the students are given opportunities to observe infant–toddler programs in the community. One center provides full day care for infants beginning at age 6 weeks and includes situationally disadvantaged children.

The director of this center is well versed in the theory and practices of the Mills College Child Life Program, and she serves on the college's infant–toddler advisory committee. Her center incorporates the "open-ended" nature of the home experience in the child care program; that is, modeling becomes the mode through which the children learn, and "clinging and following" are acceptable infant behaviors to which the adults respond. Toy selection and arrangement of the environment within age-appropriate dimensions extend the children's experiences. The students are enriched by these experiences with group care for infants and their work with these disadvantaged families.

Work with Infants in Hospitals

Group care for infants and toddlers in hospital settings provides particular challenges in that multiple caregivers including physicians, nurses, and medical technicians are a part of hospital reality. The Child Life student joins the hospital team with much detailed knowledge of the child's development, the often problematic primary relationships involved, and the responses of the patient in play. Chief among the considerations is how to provide group care for young children that is responsive to developmental needs in the context of illness and often frightening and painful experiences (Fraiberg, Shapiro, & Cherniss, 1983). Several ameliorating models are studied (Goldberger, Oremland, & Smolin, 1989).

Some students work in programs in hospitals that schedule "Infant Time" in the pediatric playroom, which is generally one hour per day when the playroom is reserved for infants and their primary caregivers. Here the student's experience at the college's infant–toddler care laboratory enables the student to create an environment conducive to play, socialization, and interaction away from medical tests and procedures. The infant and parent, when the latter is available, are encouraged to play with toys and with each other, according to responsive interactions and developmentally appropriate means, often modeled or supported by the student.

When the parents are not present, the Child Life student remains with an infant during "Infant Time." Building a play relationship that allows assessment of development and appropriate responsiveness is the basic goal. The play relationships allow for interactive play even for infants who have been secluded in a crib with medical paraphernalia and other physical restrictions.

The student conveys to the infant's nurse what the infant responds to and how this responsiveness can be continued in other relationships, decreasing the fragmentary and confusing quality that characterizes hospital relationships. At times the Child Life student extends the formal play time to become a primary person in the child's care. Concomitantly, the student frequently becomes an educator of other hospital personnel relative to infant and child development as exemplified by this student:

> During my time at the hospital, I observed many medical staff members and volunteers supporting our objectives in working with children, while others seemed only to dominate as they played or tended to engage in developmentally inappropriate play. The opportunity frequently arose in which I shared my knowledge about developmentally appropriate activities and modeled skills I had learned at the infant–toddler lab. I developed a pamphlet on the subject of working with children with limited mobility, which includes a section on infants and toddlers, and made it available to parents, volunteers, and staff.

The student further records the following two observations regarding infants:

> Tommy, a 13-month-old, was beginning to learn to walk when he was hospitalized. His mother lived a long distance away and was unable to be with him for most of his hospital stay. When the nurses were busy, Tommy was confined in his crib or in a high chair at the nurse's station. Advocating for him meant encouraging ample opportunity to practice walking, pulling up alongside furniture, and walking behind push toys. Helping the medical staff understand the importance of these experiences within the context of a consistent relationship was a major achievement.

> Shelly, a 20-month-old, was in an isolation unit. The nurses reported that they were having trouble giving oral medication. She would protest and cry. Giving her medicine became a struggle between Shelly and the nurses. Remembering the study and experience with infants and toddlers in the laboratory school, validating that children learn by exploring and interacting with their environment, I planned medical play with a doll and the medical equipment to which Shelly had been subjected. Shelly and I spent many days in such play. She was eager to perform procedures on the doll, practicing them repeatedly. Although she was preverbal, she communicated by nodding, shaking her head, and pointing. She was

obviously in control of the play, seeming bent on making sense of her own experiences.

I encouraged the nurses to give Shelly choices relative to taking the medicine. When Shelly protested on seeing the medicine, she was told that although this was the time to take the medicine, she could point to where she wanted to sit and whether she wanted to be held for the process. She could also hold the cup or have the nurse do it. Shelly took the cup, drank its contents, and with the empty medicine cup still in hand, gave the doll some medicine, too. This play with the doll continued for a number of days.

The Child Life student in their interactions with parents discuss their observations of the children and encourage the parenting relationship to continue in spite of the multiple caregivers and often intimidating setting of the hospital. This interaction parallels the parent–caregiver interactions modeled in the Mills College Children's School laboratory.

Summary

In summary, the generic underpinnings of study and work with physically well children, all of whom represent normal ranges of development and all of whom come from reasonably nurturant and functioning families, become the basis for specialty care of potentially vulnerable infants and toddlers. The Mills College Child Life Program is an example of applying basic study and experience to a special needs population.

References

Ainsworth, M., Blehar, M. C., Waters, E., & Wall, S. (1987). *Patterns of attachment.* Hillsdale, NJ: Erlbaum.

Almy, M. (1982). Applying Piaget's theory in the early childhood classroom. *Resource Reports 1982:* World Book-Child Craft.

Axtman, A. (1984). The Center for Infants and Parents at Teachers College, Columbia University: A setting for study and support. *Zero to Three, 4,* 29–34.

Bowlby, J. (1982). *Attachment and loss: Vol. 1. Attachment* (2nd ed.). New York: Basic Books.

Brazelton, T. B., & Thompson, R. H. (1988). Commentary: Child Life. *Pediatrics, 81,* 725–726.

Bronfenbrenner, U. (1979). *The ecology of human development: Experiments by nature and design.* Cambridge, MA: Harvard University Press.

Engel, G., & Reichsman, F. (1956). Spontaneous and experimentally induced depressions in an infant with a gastric fistula. *Journal of the American Psychoanalytic Association, 14,* 428–452.

Erikson, E. (1963). Play and cure. In *Childhood and Society* (pp. 222–235). New York: Norton.

Fraiberg, S., Shapiro, V., & Cherniss, D. (1983). Treatment modalities. In J. Call, E. Galenson, & R. Tyson (Eds.), *Frontiers of infant psychiatry* (pp. 56–73). New York: Basic Books.

Gaynard, L. (1990). *Psychosocial care of children in hospitals.* Washington, DC: Association for the Care of Children's Health.

Gerber, M. (1984). Caring for infants with respect: The RIE approach. *Zero to Three, 4,* 1–3.

Goldberg, S. (1982). Prematurity, effects on parent–infant interaction. In J. Belksy (Ed.), *In the beginning* (pp. 65–73). New York: Columbia University Press.

Goldberger, J. (1988). Infants and toddlers in hospitals: Addressing developmental risks. *Zero to Three, 8,* 1–6.

Goldberger, J., Oremland, E., & Smolin, A. (1989). *Child Life infant work: Do we do what we know?* Panel presentation at Child Life Council Annual Meeting, Anaheim, California.

Goldberger, J., & Wolfer, J. (1991). An approach for identifying potential threats to development in hospitalized toddlers. *Infants and Young Children, 3,* 74–83.

Gottwald, S. R., & Thurman, S. K. (1990). Parent–infant interaction in neonatal intensive care units: Implications for research and service delivery. *Infants and Young Children, 2,* 1–9.

Guillemin, J. H., & Holmstrom, L. (1986). *Mixed blessings, intensive care for newborns.* New York: Oxford University Press.

Gutkind, L. (1991). *One children's place.* New York: Penguin.

Hartley, M., White, C., & Yogman, M. W. (1989). The challenge of providing quality group child care for infants and young children with special needs. *Infants and Young Children,* 2, 1–10.

Honig, A. S., & Lally, J. R. (1981). *Infant caregiving: A design for training.* Syracuse, NY: Syracuse University Press.

The Infant Health and Development Program. (1990). Enhancing the outcomes of low-birth-weight, premature infants. *Journal of the American Medical Association, 263,* 3035–3042.

Lewis, M., & Miller, S. M. (1990). *Handbook of developmental psychopathology.* New York: Plenum Press.

Miller, K. (1993). The dual challenge: Meeting the needs of parents and babies. *Exchange, February,* 56–58.

Moss, B. (1993). From use of skills to use of self: Professional development through training to enhance relationships. *Zero to Three, 14,* 1–5.

National Center for Health Statistics. (1992, June). Number and rate of patients discharged from short stay hospitals and of days of care, and average length of stay, by age. Washington, DC: U. S. Department of Health and Human Services.

Oremland, E. (1990). Childhood illness and day care. In S. Chehrazi (Ed.), *Psychosocial issues in day care* (pp. 193–202). Washington, DC: American Psychiatric Press.

Oremland, E., & Oremland, J. (1973). *The effects of hospitalization on children.* Springfield, IL: Charles C. Thomas.

Piaget, J. (1952). *The origins of intelligence in children.* New York: International Universities Press.

Provence, S. (1989). Infants in institutions revisited. *Zero to Three, 9,* 1–4.

Richert, A. (1989, April). *The reflective practitioner.* Presentation at American Education Research Association, San Francisco.

Schulman, L. S. (1987). Knowledge and teaching: Foundations of the new reform. *Harvard Educational Review, 57,* 1–22.

Spitz, R. (1945). Hospitalism. *The Psychoanalytic Study of the Child, 1,* 53–74. New York: International Universities Press.

Torelli, L. (1989). The developmentally designed group care setting: A supportive environment for infants, toddlers and
care givers. *Zero to Three, 10,* 7–10.

Willis, W. O. (1991). Parental perspectives on the system of care
for low birth weight infants. *Infants and Young Children,
3,* v–x.

16

The Editor Responds

JEROME D. OREMLAND, M.D.

Child Life was fortunate to have Emma Plank as a founder. Clinically astute, pragmatic, and theoretically sound, Mrs. Plank developed Child Life largely from psychoanalytic theory, particularly the psychoanalytic view of trauma, the variety of responses to trauma, and the immediate and long-term consequences of trauma to development. Early on, models from social work and early childhood education were incorporated to broaden the theoretical and practice base of the emerging field. These models quickly insinuated themselves as major influences in Child Life.

Evelyn Oremland in many ways personified these developments. An experienced social worker with knowledge of psychoanalysis and with a strong background in medical sociology, she was to develop within the Department of Education at Mills College one of the first college-based Child Life programs. Her pioneering efforts fused Child Life and

211

early childhood education preparing the way for the development of Child Life as a profession.

Long concerned about the justification for Child Life programs, especially as the political and cultural medical ethos changed from support for those in need to economy of service, Dr. Oremland sought ways to show the efficaciousness of Child Life programs. Yet as noted in her introductory chapter, when it comes to hospital administrators, even quantifiable data demonstrating the economic benefits from Child Life seem to fall on deaf ears, largely because Child Life services are not directly reimbursable. Aside from justifying Child Life programs to hospital administrators, Dr. Oremland also knew the difficulties in general in demonstrating the benefits short and long term to patients. After all, prevention when effective is largely invisible.

Dr. Oremland carefully included in her teaching how various studies have demonstrated that well-established Child Life programs lessen in tangible ways the use of sedation, shorten procedure times, and directly and indirectly save medical personnel time. Yet, she knew that saving money was not what she called the essence of Child Life—dedication to decreasing the suffering of sick children and their families. Although she firmly believed that long-term prevention potentials exist in Child Life work, Dr. Oremland's focus was on the palpable ways that Child Life lessens the emotional trauma of patients and their families.

For 20 years Dr. Oremland thoughtfully read reports from her students as they performed remarkable duties in many settings with a wide variety of children. She became convinced that within these student journals lay the essence of Child Life. Her penultimate contribution to Child Life is to make these stories public and enduring.

Although the journals display a wide range of talent and inventiveness on the part of her students, the central organizing themes are few. Each story demonstrates the necessity of understanding child development; appreciating the child's way of looking at things; recognizing the role of repetition and enactment in dealing with overwhelming circumstances; being attuned to the cultural–social realities of sick children and their families; appreciating the social psychological systems within medical care; detecting the multiple interrelated effects of the child's illness within the family system; and maintaining the socializing and adapting effects of play and education.

As one would expect, Dr. Oremland begins with a discussion of play, the play partnership, and the Child Life relationship. She uses *play* in a broad sense and makes clear distinctions between play, therapeutic play, and play therapy. Quickly her discussion of the play partnership and the Child Life relationship expands to a study of the fragmentation of interpersonal experience that characterizes hospitalization. She warns that Child Life rather than unifying the hospitalized child's interpersonal experience may contribute to its fragmentation. As a specific, she warns against the ever present temptation to replace the sick child's parents, themselves absent or a detriment. Recognizing that the ideal of the single advocate and the unitary organizing personal relationship can never be achieved in a hospital, Dr. Oremland discusses ways that Child Life can counter or at least not add to the fragmenting tendencies of any child care situation.

The section "Child Life and Extended Complex Hospitalizations" represents the classical tradition of Child Life. It was out of the experiences of extended complex pediatric hospitalization that Child Life came to be. As we follow Charlie and Joel we more fully appreciate the extraordinary circumstances under which the Child Life Specialist works. Both boys had horrendous medical and socioeconomic problems, and both had severely psychologically incapacitated parents who contributed directly and enormously to their children's problems. Both children were headed for foster care placement.

Charlie particularly well illustrates how even when much medical attention is being shown, the interpersonal experience of the hospitalized child is fragmented. His rehab unit had become for him a sterile prison. His major, consistent companion was a television set over which he had no control. His extensive burn scars were frightening to other children, further contributing to his isolation.

Even though Charlie had fleeting social contacts with multiple caregivers of all levels of professional training, he had no unitary organizing interpersonal experience. Of particular concern is that Charlie became inured to the fragmentation. He protested little on being left.

Charlie's only consistent contact was with his occupational therapist (OT). Although skillful and caring, she carried the burden of having to perform painful procedures on him. Fortunately for Charlie, the medical staff recognized the need for Child Life.

The Child Life intern's visits combined with the consistent contacts with the OT became a model of knowledgeable progressive building of relationship. Using simple but consistent contact and understanding the full meaning of important interpersonal infant games, such as peek-a-boo, Kelly Nottingham gradually entered Charlie's isolation. By devising ways and with knowledgeable effort, Charlie was gradually brought to the playroom so that he could marvel at the interactions of other children and be introduced to play with other children. As Nottingham notes, "We started by wheeling him along the windows that looked into the playroom and by slowly passing the open door. We described what the kids were doing and named some of the toys. We made reassuring and encouraging comments." What Nottingham provided to this emotionally and physically scarred infant sensitively captures Dr. Oremland's essence of Child Life.

Almost unnoted is the role that Child Life played in offsetting a major psychotic symptom, Charlie's sticking his finger down his throat to induce vomiting. This severe psychiatric symptom suggests marked regressive narcissistic propensities, which the medical staff at first treated by "angry bawling out" and later by stomach intubation. With Nottingham's full-scale consistent responsiveness the symptom abated.

Joel in every way was abused. His physical injuries were severe and his psychological "hurts" profound. Rebecca Rice writes, "Because Joel was entirely dependent on others for his care, I wanted to help him gain some sense of autonomy. I decided to encourage him to name and show me medical objects. I would respond by telling him about their use."

As with Charlie, the socializing experience of the playroom was used. Even though his initial participation was from his bed, Rice notes, "Just by placing a pillow at Joel's back, he could turn enough to see the array of playroom activities. I thought (he and another child) might enjoy running drumsticks along the railings of their beds. Very quickly our corner became the band with much clanging, clacking, and jingling to be heard."

To help Joel actively master trauma, Rice introduced doll play and medical play. In the medical play, Rice took Joel's distress when his adhesive bandages were removed and turned that experience into the creative activity of "plac-(ing) tape on and then remov(ing) the tape from his (hated) restraints. The applying and removing of adhesives expanded as he was supplied with more and more sticky papers and tissue papers to exercise his newfound freedom. Eventually Band-Aids became a collage above his bed that he created."

With Joel we witness many of the striking medical reenactments of the play of medically traumatized children when given the chance. At times when the traumatic experience was too fresh, as with the anesthesia mask, Joel's play was frightened and limited. Most often he entered into play with gusto.

With great sensitivity to the medical staff's responses, Rice writes:

> As Joel became more mobile, I observed his nurses displaying more affection to him. People went out of their way to visit his room, gave him kisses, slap "high fives," or talk and play with him. It seemed that as his condition improved, everyone was less fearful of making a connection with him. . . . (W)hen survival is in question, there is a tendency for all to keep a distance.

Rice well describes the decathexis, that is, the withdrawal of emotional investment that occurs when someone is about to be lost. By decathecting the dying person, the staff members protect themselves from experiencing the loss before the loss occurs. How important it is for us to understand this defensive protective tendency to withdraw and to guard against it as best we can. Those near death more than any others need a sense of continuing investment, no matter how hard it is to maintain.

Joel's farewell party had many facets. Reflecting many student journal entries, we find the importance to the staff, often more than for the children, of parting rituals, in this case a happy one. "Joel never saw himself as the center of attention but seemed to enjoy sitting on my lap and tasting the soda and cake. . . . Eventually he chose to walk some more and the party broke up as the guest of honor strolled out the door!" Such parting rituals are important illustrations of what Dr. Oremland calls the "emotional labor" of intense involvement with sick children. Nowhere is this "emotional labor" as evident as in work with dying children.

With Charlie and Joel, the Child Life interns realized that their time with the child was limited. How much they contributed to the fragmentation of the child's interpersonal experience versus how much they organized it will depend on their success in transmitting continuations of this experience to the foster care families and the ability of these caregivers to continue it.

"Child Life and Child Death" contains among the most moving passages written on work with children. What Lauren Manheimer learned from Harry and his family is a "coming of age" study of remarkable power. In Manheimer's narrative we witness with her how ill prepared we are for life's most severe trials and the paralyzing helplessness that is often part of life. In addition, Manheimer's work is a tribute to what can be gained from respect for cultural differences and traditions. One can only marvel at the ingenuity and dedication that Manheimer manifested as she overcame a variety of procedural difficulties and traditional objections in order for this doomed child to realize what was to be one of his last wishes, to meet the tiger trainer and his animal when they visited the hospital. The drama of the event in ways eclipses how sensitively Manheimer provided the most possible within the context of the patient's circumstance, the epitome of Dr. Oremland's essence of Child Life.

Also remarkably revealed in Manheimer's and other student journals is how silently and painfully the children bear the physical distortions to their bodies that illness, medication, and surgical procedures produce. As Manheimer writes:

> On several occasions, I tried to interest Harry in coming to the playroom. . . . He repeatedly told me that he did not want to leave his room. I was concerned that Harry might be worried about how other children perceived him. After all, he was bald, attached to a number of IV lines, and needed to wear a mask. Clearly Harry did not look like an ordinary 10-year-old boy; however, in the hospital there were many children who looked like Harry, suffered similar illnesses, and felt as isolated and different from other children as he did.
>
> I was able to convince Harry to let me introduce him to another 10-year-old, African-American, hairless oncology patient. . . . The boys had much in common, played hours of

Nintendo together, and developed the beginnings of a friendship. . . .

I was successful at convincing the two boys to join me . . . in the playroom. Harry felt comfortable wearing a mask in public when he realized that (his new friend) also was required to wear one. I, too, was willing to join the group of mask-wearers for the occasion.

Dana personifies the worst fear of every parent—the well child about to enter school who seems only slightly ill and the laboratory report returns with the diagnosis of leukemia. Jacqueline McCall notes, "Dana's cancer was a new concept for . . . her family."

Dana's family from the beginning was very much a part of her hospital experience. Insisting on the importance of Dana's being at home, the mother said, "(so that she can) . . . remember who she is."

With the first recurrence of her illness, Dana's and her family's optimism gave way to bitterness and depression. Always there was the doubt that the doctors were doing all that they could. While a bone marrow transplant was being considered, Dana's illness took a turn for the worse with little hope for another remission. McCall writes, "The mother felt that Dana lost her chance for the transplant because the doctors waited in making the decision. She blamed herself for not being more aggressive."

As Dana's condition worsened, the family "guarded their time with (Dana), preferring to be alone with her. . . . Dana, too, did not ask to see people as she previously had done. . . . When the parents were not there, it was not unusual to find Dana in the corner of the playroom lying on the mat, silent and pensive." Mainly McCall would sit with her, cover her with a blanket to "make her feel cozy," and silently stroke her back.

There were long periods when Dana had little appetite, blaming the hospital food. As is frequently the case with chronically ill children, it is difficult to tell how much of

Dana's depression was due to illness, medication, or her situation. At times she would not eat or take her medications, leading to frequent, unfortunate showdowns with the medical staff.

Often Dana's family was a delight, whimsically singing and dancing with her. Yet, complex family dynamics and cultural differences made for many conflicts with the hospital staff. The mother would make lists instructing the nurses in Dana's care and isolate her from ward activities. She attempted to use the playroom to "baby-sit" Dana's siblings. The father made sexual advances to several nurses.

Dana's three siblings showed progressive evidence of the emotional toll of her illness on the family, reminding us that siblings are the unrecognized and the unserved in the havoc that chronic illness produces in families. It was heart wrenching to hear Dana's siblings on the telephone begging their mother, "Mommy, come home, come home." As one would expect, the older the child, the more specific are the manifestations of disturbance. In Dana's family, Helen, the oldest and closest to Dana, suffered the most overtly and showed profound difficulty in mourning Dana after she died. The younger brother William and the 2-year-old Dina markedly regressed. William became enuretic, and Dina showed increasingly severe separation problems with the mother.

The mother's anger over the illness took many forms. As a close relationship between Dana's mother and Child Life developed, the mother expressed angry thoughts that the hospital staff went home each night to their intact lives leaving her and her family with their problems and sorrow. One time the mother confessed to McCall, "If Dana died, it would be over. We could go on with our lives and the other kids won't have to be raised in a hospital." She spoke emotionally of having "to desert" her babies. Her statement is the closest any parent chronicled in any of the journals came to acknowledging overtly the wish that the sick child would die, although such thoughts silently permeate most of the families and staff when children are very ill over long periods of time.

Not only were the hospital and the staff the recipients of Dana's mother's anger, but her friends were as well. How disturbing it was to sense her helpless rage when at Dana's memorial service she scolded those who came to comfort her. "Where were you when I needed you? . . . You come today only for yourselves," she railed.

McCall describes the multiple roles of Child Life in dealing with Dana and her family. She attempted to maintain a consistent and soothing contact with Dana while carefully not interfering with the mother's ubiquitous presence. She absorbed much of the mother's anger and criticism, and she attempted to articulate the mother's grief, anger, and shattered hopes to her, her family, and the staff. McCall also made herself available for discussions of such painful decisions as cremation or burial.

McCall attempted to help Dana's siblings, knowing that what she could offer was limited. She noted how helpful a support group for the siblings might have been. Child Life provided the siblings some time in the playroom and some reassurance when they had difficulty with their visits, but more was obviously needed. All in all, McCall came to know the "emotional labor" of Child Life involvements as she "guard(ed) against withdrawing from (the) relationship with (a) . . . dying child" as the staff and many family members often do.

McCall's work with Dana and her family contrasts with Jo Lee's experience with Maddy, a 3-year-old infusion unit patient, and her father. Maddy's father avoided being with her during her procedures, even though he tried to make it seem that she would be less upset if he were not there. Lee tried to encourage him to remain with his daughter during her treatments or at least to tell her good-bye and that he would return. He responded by saying that she knew that he would be leaving and that he did not want her to cry. He explained, "If I stay, she cries. If I leave she doesn't." His words were diametrically opposed to what the nurses had reported—that during treatments Maddy became "rigid, screaming uncontrollably."

Lee tried to involve Maddy's father, but his apprehension overcame her best efforts. Lee returned to Maddy and with skillful reassurance and medical play, helped Maddy through the ordeal of the "push." The father remained in hiding using various rationalizations and deceptions until the procedure was over. When Maddy and her father were reunited, Maddy said, "It didn't hurt." To Lee's despair, the father responded, "I know. That's why I leave. Then she doesn't cry." Lee thought, "It is best to leave him with his idea." This is but one of many reports of how parents protect themselves from things they cannot tolerate, at times to the detriment of their children.

Although Lee's protective attitude toward the father had much to recommend it, the situation presents a dilemma common in Child Life. Although Lee helped maintain an equilibrium in the father's psychodynamics, perhaps she missed an opportunity to build a platform for future work with the father. Had Lee discussed with the father that he had much to offer Maddy and that Lee would help him more on their next visit, perhaps a new trajectory in Maddy's care might have been established.

"Child Life and Adolescents" puts into broad profile how most medical personnel come from sociological situations and life experiences very different from those of their patients. The student journals reveal the inner thoughts of young women from Mills College talking with and attempting to relate to adolescent prostitutes, girls with venereal pelvic inflammatory disease, and other young people whose lives are almost unimaginable to them. It is striking how the Child Life interns and the adolescent patients frequently find common ground and common experience, often through the youth culture, from which the students themselves are just emerging.

In "Child Life and Adolescents" the passages often are poignantly revealing of how life's ordinary issues continue even in the face of devastating and debilitating illness. One cannot help but be moved by the fact that even in the face of monumental disability and illness Amanda and Dana struggle with jealousy because Byron is more interested in one than the other. As McCall writes:

> In the playroom, Amanda sat with Dana, another preadolescent, and ate her lunch. . . . Dana told Amanda how handsome Byron was. Byron entered, and Dana, visibly happy to see him, introduced him to Amanda. Soon Byron and Dana moved to the Nintendo machine to play together. . . . Amanda stared at Byron and Dana as they played and said, "That Dana. She's just making a fool of herself . . . she has a crush on Byron". . . . She crossed her arms in front of her and watched Byron and Dana. She made faces and muttered quietly, "Oh, look at Dana go. Look at her make a fool of herself. She won't leave him alone."

In work with adolescents, the Child Life interns are confronted with a different kind of helplessness. Armed with knowledge, good intentions, and struggling with a general philosophy that love will conquer all, the students find themselves turned away by the very ones they seek to help. The conflict that Suzanne Berkes had when her coat was stolen brings into broad profile the discomfort these young women often feel when confronted with abject poverty. Berkes' sense of betrayal oscillated with self-reproach for leaving her coat temptingly unattended. Out of dedication to her profession, she decided that she and she alone had to confront Mary. It was a small but heroic act with an unexpectedly larger result. Obviously Abigail was impressed by the student's composure in the face of this challenging situation.

Clearly Abigail admired and was in awe of Berkes as she playfully mocked her. Abigail had watched Berkes closely and was amazed as she was introduced to a whole new way of dealing with people who have wronged you.

The story of Manuel, Berkes, and the book is touching. In the report we learn much about the intensity of involvement that often surrounds work with needful and appealing children. Berkes clearly had difficulty letting go of Manuel. In a sweet way the book that she made for him to help him understand his illness became her way of continuing to be with him. The book became more important to her than to Manuel. He accepted the book to help her.

Work with 12-year-old Candy presented Berkes with an order of dilemma typically not found in work with children, the evaluation of suicide and the question of confidentiality. Candy "looked well integrated. . . . She interacted easily with staff and peers . . . and had a charming sense of humor." Her demeanor was in marked contrast with her disheveled, inappropriate mother who all suspected was a drug abuser. To Berkes' surprise, while playing Scrabble with her, Candy said "that if she were on a bridge, she would probably jump from it . . . that her life was 'a mess right now.' "

Berkes knew that the comment had to be discussed with a supervisor, yet she suffered from feeling that she would be betraying Candy's trust. After some thoughtful consultation, she decided to talk with Candy about having to tell the social worker about the conversation. Instead of feeling betrayed, Berkes could sense that it was reassuring to Candy to be taken seriously and she "seemed almost grateful."

Many of the journal entries detail the ineptness of the medical staff, a blindness often stemming from ignorance and frustration. How fascinating it is to read about the young physician who thought that a challenging subjugation and intimidation would "control" Angel. His adolescent bravado led to mounting confrontation until the whole situation exploded into a frightening standoff that resulted in Angel's being physically subdued and medicated and a tension-filled ward. Angel stands out as "the failed case."

The reports also indicate how in the face of frustrating negativism, the staff may respond with regressive stubbornness. It is always astonishing to see an adult reduced to being a stubborn child by a child's frightened, defensive, negativistic stubbornness. As Janette Tacata observes:

> When I first met Lisbeth, the nursing staff was trying to have her urinate for a test. She screamed, "No! I don't want to! I want to go home! I want my Mom! You're hurting me!" I tried to comfort her, reflecting her feelings and acknowledging her discomfort. . . . Her crying became louder. She struggled with the nurses to keep from having to urinate. When they finally forced her onto the toilet seat, she continued her refusal, and the nurses became very strict with her. One said, "It doesn't matter how long you sit there. We'll sit here all day until you pee!" I could do nothing to comfort her during this standoff. I left feeling discouraged.

At times, there is clear evidence that some staff are ill suited to pediatric work. As Tacata notes:

> At one point, (Lisbeth) talked about chemo, her fear of it, and how she did not understand what it was or why she needed it. A nurse zoomed in and took over our conversation. She explained the chemo and its purpose drawing a parallel to Tide detergent and Extra-Strength Tide. I felt disregarded. When the nurse told Lisbeth she had to have chemo or die, Lisbeth became visibly upset. I tried to comfort her, but the nurse stampeded over me. Lisbeth curled up in a ball, whimpered, and went to sleep.

Time after time we see these young women skillfully and subtly educating a harassed hospital staff. Sometimes the message is simple. A little time given saves much time later. Other times the message is more complex as the Child Life intern demonstrates how establishing a relationship and providing knowledge and support can allay fears, as we see with Roberta and the laboratory technician.

Unexpectedly often the medical staff overtly allows the Child Life interns to teach them—the highest form of endorsement Child Life can receive. With Joel, Rice, "explained to the staff the importance of allowing Joel to eat with his hands permitting age-appropriate messiness. They were willing to allow . . . this even though it made more work for all involved."

Although it is easy to make villains of the medical staff, there are many tender and caring reports. What a lovely moment it was when a physician joined Kayla and Lee ("Child Life in an Infusion Unit") in reciting from C. S. Lewis.

"Child Life in the Clinics" illustrates that as medical diagnostics and treatment have expanded beyond the traditional hospital inpatient service, Child Life has moved outward into the clinics and the community. By introducing fundamental Child Life practices in a knowledgeable, caring, and sensitive way, child after child is protected from situations in which anxiety is mounting and horrible circumstances are mitigated.

Tacata's work portrays the variety of ways Child Life helps children before, during, and following frightening and painful procedures in an outpatient department. Even the "rebellious and noncompliant" Stanley, as Tacata gave words to his fears, became cooperative. As their relationship developed, Stanley was able to put more words to his unhappiness. His epithet was simple, "I hate being sick," now said and no longer acted out.

Tacata's work with Karen demonstrates how medical play in an outpatient setting can provide anticipation and reworking of frightening medical experiences, and thereby alleviate the child's distress. The exactness of detail in Karen's repetitious medical play, characteristic of medically traumatized children, vividly illustrates our understanding of turning passive into active. In her play, the acted upon becomes the actor. As the play relationship progressed, Karen's fear of crying, probably her fear of massive regression, entered her play. At a point she allowed her doll to cry and was able to comfort her.

Even though extensively prepared for a diagnostic procedure, Roberta almost came undone when something new, the machine, appeared. Adding to the tension was the technician who defensively rushed about seemingly so as not to have to relate. Yet, when the technician witnessed what skillful verbal anticipation and comforting reassurance can do, he slowed down and began to participate in the enlightened approach Tacata introduced.

Lee's experience with Lilly in an infusion unit also describes the importance of Child Life in outpatient units. Although Lilly was a "seasoned" infusion unit patient, it was upsetting to her when a new nurse attempted her transfusion without consulting Lilly about which vein to use. When the nurse failed in her attempts, tension in both patient and nurse mounted markedly. The tension increased when the nurse impatiently talked about having to use the "big needle." Fortunately, Lee knew Lilly and the procedure. She intervened, even though her intervention was not entirely welcomed by the nurse. Under a needless pressure of time, Lee fully explained that the "big needle" was essentially the same needle with which Lilly was familiar. Lee changed the emphasis by introducing the idea that the new needle was really the "blue needle." More important than the information that Lee provided Lilly was that through empathic understanding, she was able to develop a reassuring, soothing, relationship.

What followed with Lilly was surprising. Lilly began talking about having been "poked in my private parts." Lee followed up on this alarming comment and discovered that Lilly had recently had urinary catherization.

The staff was relieved by the results of Lee's work with Lilly. Seizing an opportunity to "educate" a staff that was now ready to learn, Lee discussed with staff members the importance of choice of words in work with children. These situations provided Lee with the opportunity to remind the staff how differently from adults children perceive what is said and done to them. I could not help but remember a moment that Dr. Oremland was fond of relating. One time when she was visiting a ward, a 3-year-old boy came to her and asked, "Has tomorrow come yet?" He had been promised that he could go home tomorrow.

Lee's work with 6-year-old Seb fully demonstrates medical play with reenactment and catharsis. Seb's restriction on his doll patient is especially interesting. As Lee writes, "He tore off a piece (of tape) and put it over the doll's mouth. 'I wonder why your baby needs tape over his mouth?' I asked. 'Because he screams.' he replied." His placing tape over the doll's mouth expressed his desire (to cry out angrily) and the punishment for the desire.

Skeptical hospital administrators would be pleased to learn that with Child Life on the job, only one nurse was needed to assist with Seb's procedure, not the usual four or five. Clearly we see that Child Life lessened the need for sedatives and anesthesia and all the expensive care that monitoring these medications requires. Even though Dr. Oremland would be pleased to have the skeptical hospital administrators endorse her program for these savings, silently her satisfaction would come from knowing that a child had been saved needless angst.

The Child Life interns' experiences in outpatient settings well illustrate the mounting difficulties facing patients as medical care moves toward less expensive methods of diagnosis and treatment. As fewer hospitalizations are used, more of the patient care falls to the patients themselves and their families. More and more is expected from those who have the least resources and reserves.

Lilly's grandmother in many subtle ways was resisting administering Lilly's chelation therapy at home. The staff underestimated that talking about the "pump" only frightened her. Lee thought to secure a pump and demonstrate the technique to the grandmother. Her explanation helped, but even more, "Her fear lessened when I explained a team of professionals would make home visits to help her with each step of the treatment until she felt comfortable administering the medication alone."

Danielle and her aunt also reveal the extent of the burden that is being placed on patients and their families by the new models in health care. Danielle's aunt works 7 days a week, and Danielle and she must travel a long distance by bus for Danielle's treatment for sickle cell disease. Essentially they arrive exhausted before beginning a long and difficult procedure.

On the day reported, to make matters worse, there was a long wait for a bed in the ICU. Patient and staff were running out of time and patience by the time treatment began. What followed was a nightmare of frustration, anger, and miscommunications resulting in an exhausted, frightened, sedated Danielle and a dismayed caretaker heading for home. How much more humane it could have been had Danielle been admitted the night before, renewed her contact with Lee and the nurses involved, had her treatment in the morning, and left at a time convenient for the aunt.

"Summer and the School-Age Child in the Hospital" demonstrates how bringing the Child Life orientation into traditional hospital settings can result in things being seen in new ways. Manheimer, knowing the importance of school in the social as well as cognitive development of the child, recognized that in the summer children develop many social replacements and substitutes for school allowing crucial social and cognitive development to continue—not so in the hospital. In the hospital summer and winter are the same, only in the summer there is no school program and the pediatric playroom remains largely geared for younger children. With minimal materials, Manheimer created a special space for the school-age child where socializing and cognitive activities could be maintained while school was not in session. Yet her efforts, as heroic as they were, seem a poor substitute for a child's yearning for summer. As Manheimer writes:

> It was the start of summer vacation and Harry was remembering his favorite activities in which he could not participate because of his leukemia and hospitalization. He said it was unfair. He loved the summers with the circus, feeling the sun on his back, the salty taste of seawater on his skin, the sight of children playing in the sand, and the cool sensation of ice cream dripping down his chin.

In working with drug-exposed infants and toddlers ("Child Life in a Nonhospital Setting"), Manheimer came to realize the vast limitations of the young mothers, really children themselves. The psychology of the teenage mother was fully played out. Clearly these girls often have babies hoping to take care of them the way they hoped to have been taken care of. All too often, they have babies so that they can be taken care of. In either case, crushing disappointment is inevitable.

Manheimer's observations of the mechanical way these young women dealt with their children alerted her to the fact that what was missing in their lives were tender, playful interactions between mother and child. She realized that the women were so needy and self-preoccupied that they literally "dropped off" their children and rushed to activities for themselves.

Manheimer decided that these young women needed a time to play with their children and someone to show them how to play with their children. By slowly overcoming resistances and obstacles, the play group came into being.

Manheimer's group had some disappointments, and progressively many achievements. The stories spontaneously told in the group are heartrending chronicles of social and psychological deprivations. Several of the women talked about the absence of play when they grew up; many had never had a toy. It was disturbing to observe how frequently the mothers competed with their children for attention.

Yet, there were heartwarming moments in the group when some of the young women began to see their children in new ways. It was as though they came to realize that they projected their sense of deprivation onto the children and feared these projected wishes. They came to see their children as less demanding and in that way less frightening. It was then that they spontaneously reached out to hold, love, and feel joy in playing with their infants.

Dr. Oremland's final chapter, "A Developmental Model for Training Child Life Infant Specialists for Early Intervention Programs in Hospitals and Group Care Settings," collaborated on with her colleagues and students, addresses a new interest for Child Life. Noting the increasing number of infants in the hospital, she and her Mills College colleagues developed a curriculum and practicum to equip Child Life Specialists to work with infants. On another level, the chapter presents an evolving, broadly based curriculum model for the Child Life field.

Using the Infant–Toddler Laboratory at Mills College as a complement to hospital placements, the Child Life students in this new curriculum are highly trained in normal development. The emphasis is on "child development as it is affected by illness and hospitalization, . . . (ways) to minimize the potential traumas of . . . illness and hospitalization, . . . (and on) establishing communication with the parents (so as to) integrate Child Life with family care."

In addition to the college-based multidisciplinary lectures and seminars, "debriefing" sessions after each session with the children in the laboratory are an important teaching tool integrating theory and observation. Participation in other community child care programs is used to broaden the student's knowledge of the life of the infant and the toddler. Attention is given to understanding the fragmentation of interpersonal experience that constitutes any child care situation.

Adding to the hospital internship with its journal keeping, seminars, and supervision, the mainstay of training in Child Life, is extensive experience with the "frequently bewildering and painful experiences" that constitute the infant's life in a hospital. Special attention is given to "Infant Time" in the pediatric playroom. When possible the "infant and parent . . . are encouraged to play with toys and with each other, often modeled and supported by the (Child Life) student." The play relationship is extended to the "infants who (are) secluded in a crib with medical paraphernalia and other physical restrictions."

At base, *Protecting the Emotional Development of Ill Children* is an enduring testimony to the courage and dedication of the professionals in Child Life who daily attempt to help children and their families under extraordinary circumstances. To this challenge these Child Life professionals bring their personality and the knowledge that they have worked hard to attain. These journals in particular show the influence, dedication, and gracious spirit of Evelyn Oremland, Ph.D., an extraordinary teacher who taught without so seeming. The book is an attempt to present the essence of Child Life as seen by her.

As the posthumous editor of this volume, I am grateful for the encouragement and help that I have received from the Mills College community in bringing this contribution of Dr. Oremland into being. I am especially grateful to Jo Lee, Head Teacher, Infant Toddler Program, Mills College, Oakland, California, and Kim Riemer, Child Life Specialist, University of California, San Francisco–Stanford Health Care, San Francisco, California, and Lecturer, Department of Education Child Life Program, Mills College, for their help and suggestions as I made difficult choices without having the author to guide me. Cici Oremland Teter deserves special thanks as an editor extraordinary who had the courage to improve the thinking and writing of both her father and mother.

17

Evelyn Oremland's Contributions to the Child Life Profession

KIM RIEMER, M.A.

Evelyn K. Oremland, Ph.D., Evie as she was fondly known to friends, students, and colleagues, was a passionate pioneer and visionary in Child Life. Her contributions to the field began in 1959 as the "play lady," a medical social worker assigned to the pediatric wards of the Medical Center, University of California, San Francisco, until the birth of her first child in 1961. These early years as "play lady" provided Dr. Oremland with experience with the play of hospitalized children that continued as an organizing interest throughout her professional life.

From 1961 to 1977 she devoted herself to raising her three children. In 1970 she reentered the field of Child Life by organizing a major symposium, "The Effects of Hospitalization on Children," sponsored by the Extension Division of the San Francisco Psychoanalytic Institute in cooperation

233

with the Department of Pediatrics, University of California Medical Center, Department of Pediatrics and Child Psychiatry, Stanford University Medical Center, Departments of Pediatrics and Child Psychiatry, Mt. Zion Medical Center, Department of Pediatrics, San Francisco Children's Hospital, and The Children's Hospital Medical Center of Northern California, which resulted in the book of the same name published in 1973. It was at this symposium that Dr. Oremland first met Emma Plank and began their firm and long friendship.

In 1977, Dr. Oremland founded and directed the Mills College Child Life Program, Oakland, California, the first college-based training program for Child Life Specialists on the West Coast. Her research on the effects of chronic illness and hospitalization on infants, children, and their families led to her Ph.D. in medical sociology in 1985 at the University of California, San Francisco.

The Mills College Child Life Program that she directed for over 20 years consisted of rigorous course work and practicum emphasizing the study of developmental progressions from birth to adolescence, attachment theory, mastery, the role of play in development, the effects of chronic illness and hospitalization on children and their families, and the role of the Child Life Specialist in the health care environment. The program quickly became internationally recognized.

Central to Dr. Oremland's vision of the role of the Child Life Specialist was her emphasis on teaching students how to build a therapeutic relationship with the child and his or her parents, a relationship based on acceptance, empathy, and warmth in which no expectations are placed on either child or parents. Dr. Oremland was uniquely able to combine professional knowledge with personal support for her students that provided them with an unvaryingly safe aegis under which they could develop as they struggled with the challenges of the Child Life profession.

Research was always important to Dr. Oremland. Throughout her career, she actively worked in hospital wards, playrooms, and clinics as an observer collecting clinical data for her teaching and many publications. Dr. Oremland served as consultant to The Children in Foster Care Research Project for Children's Hospital, San Francisco, California; The Child Life Program Development, Children's Hospital, Oakland, California; and Patient Care Committee, University of California Medical Center, San Francisco, California.

She was the primary researcher in Social Interactions in Growing Up with Hemophilia, University of California Medical Center, San Francisco, California; and the Playroom Observation Project, Children's Hospital, Oakland, California.

Co-editor of two books with her husband, Jerome D. Oremland, M.D., and the author of many articles, Dr. Oremland's writing elucidated the psychosocial effects of chronic illness, the problems inherent in day care with multiple caregivers, and the importance of play.

Always a close friend of such eminent leaders in Child Life and related fields as Joan and Erik Erikson, Lois Meek Stolz, and Albert J. Solnit, Dr. Oremland worked extensively to develop Child Life as a profession. From 1977 to 1979, she was Executive Board Secretary for the international organization Association for the Care of Children's Health (ACCH). From 1981 to 1996, she was a member of the Editorial Board of *Children's Health Care,* the Journal of ACCH. From 1981 to 1983 Dr. Oremland chaired the committee that developed the theoretical framework for the Child Life Council.

From 1976 to 1977 she was Vice President and from 1986 to 1988 President of the Northern California Affiliate for ACCH. From 1983 to 1984, she served as Executive Board Member of the developing international organization of the Child Life Council. As Co-Chair for the Education Committee of the Child Life Council and as a member of the Child

Life Certifying Commission from 1990 to 1992, Dr. Oremland helped develop the academic standards for Child Life professionals worldwide. In 1989 she was honored by the Child Life Council for outstanding contributions to the field.

Dr. Oremland's influence in Child Life extended beyond Mills College and the United States. She lectured in Austria, France, Israel, Italy, and Turkey. By building strong alliances with medical and academic institutions worldwide, Dr. Oremland played a critical role in expanding the Child Life field to international status, ultimately changing the way sick children and their families are cared for in medical settings throughout the world.

In 1992, Dr. Oremland lectured in Vienna on the contributions of Emma Plank and play with children in hospitals. Her eloquent paper paid tribute to the Austrian born Plank as a founder of Child Life and ignited an interest in Child Life in that country.

Believing that Child Life training serves well in a wide variety of settings for children with special needs and for agencies dealing with vulnerable children and families, in recent years Dr. Oremland encouraged her students to explore settings outside the hospital. Through her efforts, many community agencies welcomed the skills and services of the Mills College Child Life students, providing new pathways for the Child Life profession.

Dr. Oremland's career-long interest in the play of children led her to suggest a major symposium on the meaning and importance of play. Held at Mills College in 1996 to honor Dr. Oremland, the conference, "The Meaning and Significance of Play," became a memorial to her life, work, and spirit.

Dr. Oremland's colleagues, friends, and students cherished her. She was a beloved mentor and friend. As one of her students, Kelly Nottingham, said: "Few of us are fortunate enough in our lifetime to meet someone who embodies the personal qualities and professional talents we most admire. Rarely is there the opportunity to study and collaborate with such a person. I have been blessed with this experience."

Publications

Co-editor. (1973). *The effects of hospitalization on children.* Springfield, IL: Charles C. Thomas.

Co-editor. (1977). *The sexual and gender development of young children: The role of the educator.* Cambridge, MA: Ballinger.

(1985). *Social interactions in growing up with hemophilia: Developmental milestones and associated risks.* Doctoral Dissertation, University of California, San Francisco.

(1986). Communicating over chronic illness: Dilemmas of affected school aged children. *Children's Health Care, 14*(4), 218–223.

(1988). Mastering developmental and critical experiences through play and other expressive behaviors in childhood. *Children's Health Care, 16*(3), 150–156.

(1988). Work dynamics in family care of hemophilic children. *Social Science and Medicine, 26,* 467–475.

(1990). Childhood illness and day care. In S. Chehrazi (Ed.), *Psychosocial issues in day care* (pp. 193–202). Washington, DC: American Psychiatric Press.

(1993). Abreaction. In C. E. Schaefer (Ed.), *The therapeutic powers of play* (pp. 143–165). Northvale, NJ: Jason Aronson.

Presentations

(1966, Spring). Bringing child development perspectives to pediatrics. U.S. Air Force Hospital, Department of Pediatrics, Ankara, Turkey.

(1968, January). Play programs for pediatric services. Community Mental Health Center, Salt Lake City.

(1968, Spring). Understanding children's play. Children's Clinic of Dr. Frijling Schreuder, Amsterdam.

(1973, Summer). The effects of hospitalization on children. University of Washington Hospital, Family Medicine Clinic, Seattle.

(1973, Summer). Adding new dimensions to pediatric care. Children's Memorial Hospital, Omaha.

(1974, January). Listening to children in pediatric care. Primary Children's Hospital, Salt Lake City.

(1974, Spring). Teaching pediatric staffs about children's play. Child Guidance Clinic, Children's Hospital, San Francisco.

(1975, Spring). Interactions with children in health care. Pediatric Grand Rounds, Children's Hospital, San Francisco.

(1975, Spring). Psychological development in children through pediatric care. Child Welfare League of America, San Diego.

(1976, Spring). Minimizing developmental disruptions for children in hospitals. American Association of Psychiatric Services for Children, San Francisco.

(1976–1978). Adapting social work with young children in pediatric care. School of Social Welfare, University of California, Berkeley. Spring sessions.

(1976, January). Developmental progressions through children's play. Northern California Affiliate, Association for the Care of Children's Health, San Francisco.

(1977, Fall). Child development perspectives for work in P. T. Department of Physical Therapy, University of California, San Francisco.

(1978, April). Responses of children to illness. Northern California Chapter, National Association for the Education of Young Children, San Jose, California.

(1978, Fall). Academic content for pediatric staffs. Department of Medical Psychology, University of California, San Francisco.

(1979, October). Enhancing nursing care on pediatrics. Acute Care Pediatric Nurse Conference. Children's Orthopedic Hospital, Seattle.

(1979, June). *Education and training issues for Child Life workers: What is the ideal?* Panel presentation, Annual Meeting of the Association for the Care of Children's Health, Los Angeles.

(1980, Spring). *What special children need.* Panel discussion, California State Education Commission on Young Children with Exceptional Needs, San Francisco.

(1980, April). The development of a new profession for work with children. American Education Research Association, Boston.

(1980, July). Spontaneous, traumatic play—Another dimension of work with children. Annual Meeting of the Association for the Care of Children's Health, Dallas.

(1980, November). Bringing knowledge of children's play to pediatrics. National Association for the Education of Young Children, San Francisco.

(1982, June). Considerations of disease uniqueness as an influence in development. Annual Meeting of the Association for the Care of Children's Health, Seattle.

(1985, July). Symbolic representations in the play of sick children. Hadassah Hospital, Jerusalem.

(1985, October). Meanings in children's play—Emma Plank's contribution. Vienna.

(1986). Sick child care in day care: Meeting the needs of parents and children in a changing society. Workshop leader, San Francisco.

(1988, June). *Emotional labor in Child Life Work.* Panel presentation. Annual Meeting of the Child Life Council, Cleveland.

(1989, May). *Do we do what we know? Work with infants in hospitals.* Panel presentation. Annual Meeting of the Child Life Council, Anaheim.

(1990). Selecting literature for Child Life training and staff development. Annual Meeting of the Child Life Council, Washington, DC.

(1992, May). Achieving excellence in supervision. Annual Meeting of the Child Life Council, Atlanta.

(1992, Fall). The contributions of Emma Plank and play with children in hospitals. University Hospital, Vienna.

(1993, May). Child Life abroad. Annual Meeting of the Child Life Council, Chicago.

(1994, May). Panel on *Child Life internships*. Annual Meeting of the Child Life Council, Toronto.

(1995, October). Motherhood—Myths and realities. Chair. Mills College, Oakland, California.

Postscript

Cost Effectiveness and Child Life

Kim Riemer, M.A.

Without question Dr. Evelyn Oremland's foremost interest was in the alleviation of needless sadness, anguish, pain, apprehension, and fear, and in the protection of the emotional development of children. Her students' journals vividly testify support for the research that demonstrates the effectiveness of psychological preparation of hospitalized children in reducing anxiety and in enhancing coping (Wolfer, Gaynard, Goldberger, Laidley, & Thompson, 1988). Less anxious, more cooperative children directly translate into time savings for the medical staff, which of course means financial savings for the hospital. Clearly, medical staff have limited time and theoretical knowledge for the type of in-depth psychological preparation from which hospitalized children benefit most.

241

Yet today, only 15% of the 3 million children hospitalized each year are served by medical facilities that have Child Life programs (American Academy of Pediatrics, 1998). Although the American Academy of Pediatrics (1993) recommended that hospitals retain at least one Child Life Specialist for pediatric patients and the Joint Commission on Accreditation of Health Care Organizations includes Child Life services in its review matrices of the 4,000 hospitals in the United States and Canada that have child patients, a mere 400 hospitals maintain Child Life programs (Child Life Council, 1996a, 1996b, 1997). Only New Jersey has placed a requirement for Child Life services in its "Hospital Licensing Standards" (New Jersey *Register*, 1989).

The Phoenix Children's Hospital Research Project, supported by the Association for the Care of Children's Health, has become the model demonstration that children admitted for surgical procedures show better physical recovery, need less sedation and narcotics, and require fewer days of hospitalization (Gaynard, Wolfer, Goldberger, Thompson, Redburn, & Laidley, 1990). The Phoenix project has shown that developmentally sensitive preparation of children frequently results in child patients who require minimal physical restraint by hospital staff and reduced sedation and analgesics with the costly monitoring that these medications require.

These direct benefits from Child Life services, however, at times eclipse other fiscal benefits. For example, children typically regress after leaving the hospital. Part of the Child Life Specialist's work is to prepare the parents for these eventualities and to provide ways for parents and caregivers to support the child during difficult transitions. This fuller type of discharge planning that characterizes Child Life work increases the success of patient care at home, potentially decreasing noncompliance and costly rehospitalizations (Thompson & Stanford, 1981).

Experience reveals the *cost effectiveness* (not to mention the emotional distress saved the staff) of Child Life programs, the cost of which is minimal. Salaries comprise 87% of the cost of Child Life programs, and Child Life Specialists by hospital standards, or by any standard, are not a weighty expenditure. The average entry-level salary of a Child Life Specialist in the late 1990s is low (Snow & Triebenbacher, 1994).

A less heralded advantage of Child Life Programs is their striking public appeal. Child Life promotes "satisfied consumers." Knowledgeable parents increasingly want to know the kinds of psychological support that will be available to their child and themselves during hospitalization. Also seeing children, despite their heavy medicosurgical incumbencies, playing actively in attractive playroom settings can provide fund-raising opportunities.

Currently Child Life services are not reimbursable. This is a complicated matter. Many Child Life professionals are reluctant to press for direct charges for Child Life services, even as specific as presurgical preparation. Direct charge for Child Life services might result in some children being deprived of the service if they are not on the proper reimbursement plan.

Clearly hospital administrators need continuing enlightenment, and patients and their families must make their wishes known regarding psychosocial programs. Although always guided by a desire to reduce suffering, and despite a remarkable ability to develop a cadre of devoted workers, Oremland knew, as chronicled in her history of children in the hospital, that major changes in pediatric care primarily come with governmental sanctions. As always, children, be they sick or well, need advocacy from powerful political allies.

References

American Academy of Pediatrics, Committee on Hospital Care: Child Life Programs. (1993). *Pediatrics, 91,* 671–673.

American Academy of Pediatrics, Committee on Hospital Care. (1998). Policy statement. *Pediatrics, 101,* 671–673.

Child Life Council. (1996a). *Directory of Child Life Programs in North America.* Rockville, MD: Author.

Child Life Council. (1996b). *Committee Report on Joint Commission of Accreditation of Health Care Organizations, America.* Rockville, MD: Author.

Child Life Council. (1997). *Guidelines for the Development of Child Life Programs.* Rockville, MD: Author.

Gaynard, L., Wolfer, J., Goldberger, J., Thompson, R., Redburn, L., & Laidley, L. (1990). *Psychosocial Care of Children in Hospitals. Clinical Practice Manual from the Child Life Research Project.* Washington, DC: Association for the Care of Children's Health.

New Jersey *Register.* (1989). Monday, September 18, CITE 21, 2925–2949.

Snow, C., & Triebenbacher, S. (1994). *Child Life employment trends and practices.* Presented at the Annual Conference of the Association for Care of Children's Health, Toronto.

Thompson, R., & Stanford, G. (1981). *Child Life in hospitals.* Springfield, IL: Charles C. Thomas.

Wolfer, J., Gaynard, L., Goldberger, J., Laidley, L., & Thompson, R. (1988). An experimental evaluation of a model Child Life program. *Children's Health Care, 16,* 244–254.

Glossary

ACQUIRED IMMUNE DISEASE SYNDROME (AIDS) A chronic, usually lethal, viral disease that suppresses the immune system resulting in progressive, overwhelming infections. AIDS is transmitted by intimate contact, contaminated needle contact, and contact with contaminated blood, in the past via blood transfusion.

ACUTE LYMPHOCYTIC LEUKEMIA (ALL) A cancer of the white blood cells of the body often referred to as childhood leukemia because it most frequently affects children.

ACUTE MYELOGENOUS LEUKEMIA (AML) A rapidly invasive cancer of the white blood cells produced by the bone marrow.

APLASTIC ANEMIA A severe form of anemia in which the body stops making new blood cells. Often requires blood transfusion.

APPENDICITIS Acute inflammation of the appendix, a part of the large intestine. Usually requires surgery.

BLOOD TRANSFUSION The administering of blood via intravenous infusion.

245

BONE MARROW BIOPSY A surgical procedure in which small pieces of bone marrow tissue are taken for microscopic study.

BROVIAC An intravenous catheter placed into a large vein of the body.

CATHERIZATION The introduction of a small flexible catheter. Catheters are introduced into the bladder to drain the bladder for tests, to introduce medications, or to relieve obstructions. Catheters are also introduced into veins through needles to obtain blood or to introduce medications.

CENTRAL LINE Intravenous catheter placed into larger veins of the body.

CHEMOTHERAPY (CHEMO) Medications for treating cancer.

CYSTIC FIBROSIS A common, fatal genetic disease in which the internal ducts of the organs of the body, especially the lungs, are blocked with thick mucus.

DESFERRAL A drug administered to dissipate the accumulation of iron in frequently blood-transfused patients.

DIABETES MELLITUS A condition, sometimes hereditary, in which there is a lack in ability to metabolize blood glucose.

ENURESIS Loss of bladder control in a child previously bladder trained, or in an adult.

EWING'S SARCOMA A malignant tumor of the bone.

GASTRIC TUBE A plastic tube inserted through the nose or mouth into the stomach for feeding and/or the introduction of medication.

HEMATOLOGY The study of blood.

HUMAN IMMUNODEFICIENCY VIRUS (HIV) The virus causing AIDS.

IMMUNOSUPPRESSED A condition in which the immune system is compromised either by illness or medications, lessening the body's ability to fight off infections.

INTENSIVE CARE UNIT (ICU) A specialized unit for close monitoring of critically ill patients.

INTRAVENOUS BOARD (IV BOARD) A small piece of plastic attached to the patient with adhesive tape at the site of an intravenous infusion to restrict movement so as not to disturb the flow of the infusion.

INTRAVENOUS INFUSION (IV) A flexible catheter with a needle placed in the vein to inject medicines or replace fluids. The infusion often takes hours, and the canisters containing the fluids are attached to IV poles, sometimes called "trees." During an IV, the patient is only somewhat mobile depending on the capability of moving the pole.

INTRAVENOUS STICKS (IV STICKS) The insertion of the needle into the vein to begin an intravenous infusion or to withdraw blood for tests. At times, it is difficult to insert the needle (commonly called "finding" the vein), and several "sticks" may be required.

LUMBAR PUNCTURE (LP) A procedure that entails the insertion of a needle under local anesthesia into the lumbar region of the back between the vertebrae to the membrane sac that surrounds the brain and spinal cord. The procedure is diagnostic when cerebrospinal fluid is withdrawn for study. It can also be a way of introducing medication into the cerebrospinal fluid.

LUPUS (SYSTEMIC LUPUS ERYTHEMATOSUS [SLE]) A disease of unknown origin in which inflammatory lesions involve many body systems.

MEDICAL PLAY Children's play using actual medical equipment or toy representations of apparatus used in hospitals for patient treatment. In the play, the child often spontaneously assumes the role of doctor, nurse, or health care professional and uses dolls as patients to reenact actual procedures or the child's fantasies of procedures that they have or will experience.

METASTASIS (METS) A malignant growth that develops from the spread of abnormal cells from the cancer of origin.

MORPHINE A narcotic and analgesic medication typically used for patients in extreme pain.

NARCOTICS ANONYMOUS (NA) A self-help group patterned after Alcoholics Anonymous to help individuals overcome drug addiction.

NEUTROPENIC A condition resulting in a low white blood cell count that leaves the body unable to fight infection.

ONCOLOGY The study of cancers.

PARAPLEGIC The condition of being paralyzed from the waist down.

PELVIC INFLAMMATORY DISEASE (PID) An infection, usually venereal, of the ovaries, Fallopian tubes, and/or uterine lining.

PROPHYLACTIC A preventive medicine or procedure.

REHABILITATION (REHAB) A phase in medical treatment that focuses on the whole patient to enable him or her to reachieve the fullest functioning following an accident or illness. Hospitals often have special units called rehabilitation or rehab units.

SEIZURE A sudden convulsion resulting from infection, fever, trauma, or other abnormalities of the brain.

SICKLE CELL ANEMIA A genetic blood disease in which the red blood cells change from round to sickle shape, making free flow of blood in the blood vessels difficult. The disease is most frequently found in America among African Americans.

SPINA BIFIDA A congenital condition that results from the incomplete closure of the lower part of the spinal column.

TOTAL EXCHANGE The exchange of a large amount of diseased blood, usually during a sickle cell episode, with an equal amount of new blood.

TRACHEOTOMY A surgical opening made into the wind-pipe through the neck to assist respiration and keep airways unobstructed.

VASO-OCCLUSIVE EPISODE Clogging of the free flow of blood in the arteries and veins of the body. If in the brain, "strokes" may occur. In sickle cell disease, vaso-occlusive episodes are frequent and painful.

Index

251